BLUEPRINTS
USMLE Step 2 CS

BLUEPRINTS
USMLE Step 2 CS

Carter E. Wahl, MD
Resident in Pathology
University of California San Diego
San Diego, California

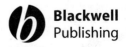
Blackwell
Publishing

Copyright © 2005 by Carter E. Wahl, MD 2005

Blackwell Publishing, Inc., 350 Main Street, Malden, Massachusetts 02148-5018, USA
Blackwell Publishing Ltd, 9600 Garsington Road, Oxford OX4 2DQ, UK
Blackwell Publishing Asia Pty Ltd, 550 Swanston Street, Carlton, Victoria 3053, Australia

04 05 06 07 5 4 3 2 1

ISBN: 1-4051-0445-7

Wahl, Carter E.
  Blueprints USMLE step 2 CS / Carter E. Wahl.
      p. ; cm.
  Includes bibliographical references and index.
  ISBN 1-4051-0438-4 (pbk.)
  1. Physicians–Licenses–United States–Examinations–Study guides. 2. Clinical
medicine–Examinations, questions, etc.
  [DNLM: 1. Medicine–Problems and Exercises. 2. Educational Measurement. W 18.2
W146b 2005] I. Title: USMLE step 2 CS. II. Title: Blueprints USMLE step two CS.
III. Title.

  R834.5.W34 2005
  610'.76–dc22

                                   2004017582

A catalogue record for this title is available from the British Library

Acquisitions: Beverly Copland
Development: Selene Steneck
Production: Jennifer Kowalewski
Cover design: Hannus Design Associates
Interior design: Mary McKeon, revised by Shawn Girsberger
Typesetter: International Typesetting and Composition in India
Printed and bound by Walsworth Publishing in Marceline, MO

For further information on Blackwell Publishing, visit our website:
www.blackwellmedstudent.com

Notice: The indications and dosages of all drugs in this book have been recommended in
the medical literature and conform to the practices of the general community. The medications described do not necessarily have specific approval by the Food and Drug
Administration for use in the diseases and dosages for which they are recommended. The
package insert for each drug should be consulted for use and dosage as approved by the
FDA. Because standards for usage change, it is advisable to keep abreast of revised recom-
mendations, particularly those concerning new drugs.

The publisher's policy is to use permanent paper from mills that operate a sustainable
forestry policy, and which has been manufactured from pulp processed using acid-free
and elementary chlorine-free practices. Furthermore, the publisher ensures that the text
paper and cover board used have met acceptable environmental accreditation standards.

For Matthew G. Wahl and Kathryn E. Wahl

Contents

Reviewers . . . .*ix*

Preface . . . .*xi*

Note to Readers . . . .*xiii*

1 Description of the Step 2 CS 1

2 Exam Development 3

3 The Standardized Patient 5

4 The Day of the Test 7

5 Seeing Your Patients 10

6 Atypical Cases 27

7 Style and Grace 31

8 Scoring 34

9 Practice Cases 37

References *141*

Index *143*

Reviewers

Katharine Fast, MD
Intern
Stanford University Medical Center
Palo Alto, California

David Gloss, MD
1st year resident, Medicine/Neurology
Tulane University
New Orleans, Louisiana

Rebecca Guinn
Class of 2005
Texas Tech University Health Sciences Center
Lubbock, Texas

Shane LaRue
Class of 2005
Medical College of Wisconsin
Milwaukee, Wisconsin

Azam Mohiuddin
Class of 2005
University of Kentucky
Lexington, Kentucky

Benjamin W. Sears
Class of 2005
Loyola University Chicago Stritch School of Medicine
Maywood, Illinois

Preface

This book provides a review of the USMLE Step 2 CS to help ensure that you pass the first time. There is a wealth of detailed information about the exam including scheduling, eligibility, and other logistical information on the USMLE website (http://www.usmle.org). This book is not a recapitulation of the website, and you should still read and understand the information there. To limit your study time and ensure you pass the first time, continue reading. The following is a brief description of each chapter:

Chapter 1—Description of the Step 2 CS provides an overview of the basic exam structure including the format, the types of cases you will likely encounter, and how the test is administered. This chapter is intended to provide a basic outline of the exam. Much more information about the exam structure is available on the USMLE website (www.usmle.org).

Chapter 2—Exam Development discusses the purpose of the exam and how diseases and clinical skills were selected for the test to best fulfill the purpose. By learning how the test was developed you can anticipate the types of cases you can expect to see on the exam and prepare accordingly.

Chapter 3—The Standardized Patient provides a description of standardized patients including how they are trained and how they evaluate you. By understanding these patients you will know how they view you and how you can optimize your interaction with them.

Chapter 4—The Day of the Test provides a picture of the exam day and practical information about getting to the test center, what to bring, and what to wear so you arrive prepared and relaxed.

Chapter 5—Seeing Your Patients provides a detailed discussion about interacting with your patients in the typical case. The typical case is one requiring you to take a history, perform a physical exam, communicate with your patient, and write a patient note. A strategy for the entire encounter including an easy-to-remember plan for each step is provided.

Chapter 6—Atypical Cases addresses those cases that don't follow the typical case format. Such cases need to be approached somewhat differently. Atypical case topics are discussed along with possible approaches to these patients.

Chapter 7—Style and Grace discusses several commonly occurring difficult situations that may arise because the exam is a timed simulation with acting that is generally awkward. This chapter provides suggestions for handling the difficult situations gracefully.

Chapter 8—Scoring discusses how your skills will be evaluated. This exam is scored differently than others and understanding the scoring process is essential for superior performance, and it will help streamline your review.

Chapter 9—Practice Cases provides several cases with patient introductions and case objectives similar to those on the actual exam. Sample checklists and patient notes are provided so you can practice and monitor your performance.

Note to Readers

Over the years, testing methods in education have evolved in an attempt to arrive at a format that optimizes a number of variables including reliability, validity, cost, and overall ease of administering medical training exams. In the medical field, where the knowledge and skills of effective practitioners change, the definition of an appropriate exam changes too. Until about 50 years ago, exams in medical education were mostly in oral and essay form. These formats accurately assess an examinee's knowledge, but they are somewhat limited by inconsistent scoring, excessive time to administer, and their inability to cover a broad range of topics.

Because they can be scored consistently and they can cover a lot of material in a short time, multiple-choice exams have become the preferred format. Multiple-choice exams have their own limitations. They have artificial prompts that allow guessing, and they deviate significantly from the way knowledge is applied in most real-world settings. An objective way of assessing clinical skills that combines the strengths of the more traditional exam formats has been sought for years. In the 1970s, the OSCE (Objective Structured Clinical Exam) was born.

The OSCE is an exam where the test-taker goes through a series of stations, each with a standardized clinical task that needs to be completed. An observer at each station has a checklist of predetermined appropriate actions. Scores are assigned based on the number of checks an examinee receives. The exam format is without the artificial prompts of multiple-choice and the checklist, which is hidden from the examinee during the test, provides a level of objectivity. The multitude of stations allows coverage of a sufficient range of material. This exam format has been found effective in a number of settings including dentistry, medicine, and physical therapy. Its strengths and limitations have been thoroughly studied. In 1998, a version of the OSCE called the Clinical Skills Assessment (CSA) was required of foreign medical graduates wishing to practice in the United States. The exam proved to be an accurate assessment of medical knowledge and communication skills. The National Board of Medical Examiners developed an OSCE that is similar to the CSA and it became part of the USMLE Step 2 exam in June of 2004. It is called the USMLE Step 2 Clinical Skills or USMLE Step 2 CS.

1 Description of the Step 2 CS

The exam is designed to closely mimic the typical clinic day of a practicing physician. The setting is a medical clinic with multiple exam rooms stocked with the basic medical supplies you would need to perform a physical exam. The test consists of 12 rooms or stations. You will start at one room and rotate through the entire course. There will be others taking the exam simultaneously, rotating through the rooms ahead and behind you as you go. Each examinee will be assigned a starting room. When testing begins, you will be positioned in front of the closed door to your first station. A brief written description of the patient and the objectives for the visit will be posted on the door for you to read. The objective for each station may be somewhat different.

■ THE TYPICAL STATION

The typical station consists of a patient who has a medical problem. Your objective will be to take the patient's history and perform a physical exam. Depending on the case, you may be asked to take a partial history and perform a focused physical exam. During your visit you will be evaluated on your ability to communicate and establish rapport with the patient, elicit a history, and perform a physical exam. After your visit, you will have to write a brief note about your encounter including your differential diagnosis, history and physical exam findings, and a diagnostic work-up. Most cases will follow this general format.

■ OTHER POSSIBLE SITUATIONS

Some stations may have different objectives. You may have a drug-seeking patient, a victim of abuse, or a patient seeking absence from work. These more socially-oriented cases may not require a physical exam, but instead will ask you to interact with the patient in some way that will test your decision-making and communication skills. Other cases may only indirectly involve a patient. For example, you may have a telephone conversation with a patient in which the patient describes a problem and you have to assess the urgency of the situation and make a plan. There are no pediatric cases on the exam, but you may encounter a parent with questions about his or her child. You may have an ECG or x-ray to interpret and describe to a patient. You may have a case with a plastic model or other patient simulator to perform a maneuver that is otherwise not allowed, such as a breast exam. You may even have a case that is being tested for future use. These cases will not be part of your final score, and you will not know which ones, if any, they are. In short, cases can take a number of forms and each assesses different skills.

■ THE PATIENT ENCOUNTER

Cases involving a patient will have a standardized patient who is a healthy person that has been trained to respond to your questions or physical exam in a way that portrays a specific illness or problem. The patient will have checklists of predetermined items that represent an ideal interaction. The typical cases may have two checklists. One checklist represents the ideal history, and the other represents the ideal physical exam for that case. You cannot see the checklists while you are with the patient, and the patient will fill them out after your visit is over. You will be timed during each case, and warnings will be given a few minutes before time expires with your patient and again before time expires for your note writing. You will have 15 minutes to see your patient and 10 minutes to write your note. There are a variety of case types and patient problems, and the exact requirement for each station will be stated in the posted objectives that you read before seeing the patient.

2

Exam Development

The purpose of the exam is to assess your ability to perform a history and physical exam, consider possible diagnoses, and effectively communicate with your patient. The exam content and format were developed in a way that would best measure these skills. Understanding the examination design will help you know what is expected of you and how you can best prepare.

■ EXAM BLUEPRINTS

Because of the number of people taking the test, the examiners needed a large pool of testable items that would allow variation in the content from one testing session to the next and still measure test takers' skills equally and effectively. An examination blueprint was developed to achieve this goal. The examination blueprint determines what illnesses are testable, what clinical skills are testable, and how they can be combined into a clinical encounter to assess an examinee's skill level. Examination blueprints were established in the following way:[1]

Testable clinical situations were determined by sending a large list of health problems to experienced practicing physicians and students whose skills were of the level being tested. The students were asked to rank the illnesses by how often they encountered them, and the experienced physicians were asked to rank them subjectively by their importance in medical education. Illnesses ranked highly by both groups were then checked against how common they were in several large medical facilities. Items ranking highly by all three methods were considered important, common, and therefore testable. Another list containing clinical skills such as history taking, performing a physical exam, clinical reasoning, and patient education was similarly assessed. The result was two lists, one of common and important clinical problems and one of common and important clinical skills. The blueprint is a combination of the lists. Items from each list could be paired to make an examination case topic. In this way a large number of testable situations that are considered equal assessments of a student's ability were established, eliminating the need to repeat the exact same examination for all test-takers. A sample blueprint is shown below:

	Cardiovascular	Neurology	Gastrointestinal	Psychiatric
Physical exam				
History				
Communication				

The real blueprint is much larger. By selecting any empty box, the examiners choose a case topic and clinical skill to be assessed for any given administration of the exam with assurance that one selection is as challenging and as good of an assessment of student performance as another. In the above blueprint, a case requiring a physical exam for a cardiovascular problem is as testable as a case requiring a history for a psychiatric problem. The illnesses are generalized into organ system or body region and not by diagnosis because USMLE Step 2 CS patients generally don't require a specific diagnosis. Instead, the test taker must provide a differential diagnosis.

Because of the way the blueprint was created, you can assume you will have cases encompassing a variety of organ systems that represent commonly occurring medical complaints. The medical examiners have emphasized the following broad categories as likely exam topics: constitutional symptoms, cardiovascular, gastrointestinal, genitourinary, musculoskeletal, neurological, psychiatric, respiratory, and women's health.[2] You can also assume that you will be required to perform a variety of common clinical tasks. Examples include taking a history and performing a physical exam, clinical decision-making, and note writing. Rare diseases and unusual or sophisticated procedures are unlikely to be part of the exam. Therefore, you can focus on practicing and refining the knowledge and skills you use most often.

3 The Standardized Patient

The standardized patients are healthy people who have been trained to realistically portray an illness or problem. They have the dual function of simulating a patient and evaluating you. Standardized patients are specifically trained in:

Patient simulation, including:

- Responding to your questions in a consistent, predetermined way
- Simulating specific symptoms and physical exam findings
- Portraying patient subtleties including affect, body language, etc.
- Asking you relevant questions
- Not leading or inhibiting you in any way
- Ensuring consistency among examinees

Evaluation, including:

- Assessing your verbal and nonverbal communication skills
- Assessing your grasp of the English language
- Noting what parts of the physical exam you performed
- Assessing your physical exam technique
- Assessing your overall character including mood and level of interest
- Completing checklists for scoring

For an exam that uses standardized patients to be a functional measurement of student performance it is imperative that the patients are trained to be realistic, consistent, and adhere strictly to their training during the exam. Standardized patient encounters have become a routine part of clinical training, and the making of a standardized patient has become a well-defined process with strict requirements. To ensure peak performance, standardized patients go through an intense training program.

A multitude of books and training courses are available to ensure that patients are trained in a way that makes them truly standardized. Training for standardized patients generally involves a detailed one-on-one session with a person who is experienced with the clinical situation that is to be portrayed. Patients are selected to portray a case because they meet certain physical features such as age, height, weight, etc., and they demonstrate the ability to accurately simulate the condition being tested. Patients are coached on every detail about the case including appropriate body language, eye contact, and affect.

The goal of training is to provide the standardized patient with medical knowledge that is comparable to that of a real patient with the disease. With proper training, standardized patients can portray a disease with accuracy, reproducibility, and versatility that approaches that of a real patient.[3] Because standardized patients will evaluate you, you may find it beneficial to learn more about their training and how they are taught to view you. For more information you can consult the following sources:

The website of the Association of Standardized Patient Educators at: http://www.aspeducators.org/sp_info.htm.

Barrows, Howard S. *Training Standardized Patients to Have Physical Findings*. Southern Illinois University, School of Medicine, 1999.

Barrows, Howard S. *Simulated (Standardized) Patients and Other Human Simulations*. Health Sciences Consortium, Chapel Hill NC, 1987.

You do not need to become an expert in standardized patient education to do well on the exam. But it is important to understand that standardized patients receive extensive training. They are carefully selected for their skills and need to be taken seriously. *A standardized patient's actions and responses all have meaning. You should never assume that a subtle physical attribute or speech irregularity represents some flaw of the real person portraying the patient.* Alternatively, you should never assume that some aspect of the history or physical exam can be ignored because the patient is not real. In short, pay attention to your standardized patients. They are trying to tell you something.

4 The Day of the Test

You will be given an orientation immediately before the exam begins. Test center staff will be present during the exam to answer your questions and ensure that you are in the right place. You will be given plenty of instruction, and there are steps you can take before exam day to ensure you get the most out of it.

■ FAMILIARIZE YOURSELF WITH THE EXAMINATION PROCESS

Though you will be given an orientation, you should have some basic understanding of the exam before you arrive. Hopefully, you have had experience with a standardized patient exam sometime before the USMLE Step 2 CS. Having prior experience is beneficial, but you must remember that each exam is somewhat different and the rules for the USMLE version may be different from what you have experienced before. It is up to you to know and abide by the rules for the USMLE. The following facts will help familiarize you with the USMLE version. You should also review the USMLE website (http://www.usmle.org) for the official exam instructions.

■ ARRIVE EARLY

Because you are taking the exam alongside others, the orientation and exam will start on time with or without you. If you arrive late you may miss the orientation or be required to reschedule the exam altogether (with a fee). You may be taking the test in an unfamiliar city and you may want to arrive a day or so early and locate the test center before the morning of the exam. If possible, stay near the test center, as traffic and travel time may be unfamiliar to you.

■ DRESS WELL AND LOOK PROFESSIONAL

You will be seeing a number of different people who will be evaluating you based on brief encounters. Whether it is fair or not, your appearance will play a major role in your standardized patients' first impression and overall assessment of you. It is to your advantage to look your best. Make sure your clothing is appropriate and clean. Do not wear excessive jewelry. Have clean and neat appearing hands. In short, look professional.

TRAVEL LIGHT

You should bring only the following items with you to the test site:

- A clean white lab coat (note clean!)
- A stethoscope
- A watch
- Your driver's license or passport
- Your scheduling permit (the name must exactly match the name on your identification)
- A snack and lunch (a light meal is provided if you forget)

You do not need to bring anything else with you, especially a cell phone, pager, or personal digital assistant (PDA) that you will have to store during the exam. Before entering the test center, empty your white coat of all pocket cards, books, or other aids commonly used when seeing real patients. Such things are prohibited and being caught with them during the exam may be considered cheating. You will be given a small, unsecured space to store other items you may have, but it is probably easiest to bring just the essentials. Wear a watch so you can monitor time during your cases. Be aware that excessive concern with time or using a watch with an alarm may be disruptive to your patients and viewed negatively by them.

WARM UP

Having to wake up on exam day and immediately begin reading, writing, communicating, and meeting people can be difficult. After the exam most test-takers feel like they did their best on the middle 6 or 8 stations, after they have warmed up but before fatigue sets in. Though you may not be able to eliminate fatigue at the end of the day, you will have a significant advantage on the first few cases by warming up prior to the exam. Get a newspaper and force yourself to read and process information before the test. Critically read an article or interpret a graph in the business section to sharpen your mind. On most days, people don't have to perform right away in the morning as they must on exam day. You may be unpleasantly surprised if the introduction to the first patient is the first thing you critically read on exam day.

▇ EXAM STRUCTURE

Your day will begin with the orientation. Again, remember that the instruction and rules outlined during the orientation are to be followed and may differ from your past experience with standardized patient examinations. During the orientation you will learn the following general rules:

- The exam takes about 8 hours in addition to the orientation time.
- You are allowed 2 breaks during the test.
- You may not discuss the exam with anyone at any time during the test or the breaks or anytime after the exam.
- No one is to speak in any language but English, even during breaks.
- Once you enter the test center you may not leave until you complete the exam.
- You may not use a cell phone, even during breaks.

The basic exam structure is as follows:

- A starting station will be assigned.
- You will be given time to read a brief description of the patient and the objectives for that case.
- You may then enter the room with the patient where you must complete the objectives. *You will have 15 minutes for the patient visit.*
- A buzzer or a knock on the door will warn you a few minutes before your time with the patient expires.
- The standardized patient will ask you to stop when time is up.
- When you leave your patient you will *not* be allowed to go back and see him or her *for any reason.*
- *You will be given 10 minutes to write a note about your patient encounter.*
- You will then move to the next station and repeat the above process. There are 11–12 stations in total.
- All stations are video recorded.

With preparation, the above process can be completed efficiently and effectively. Again, some cases may have a different format or objective. The features of a typical case will be discussed individually in greater detail in Chapter 5, Seeing Your Patients.

5 Seeing Your Patients

The following description assumes that all cases will follow the standard format, which includes taking the patient's history, performing the physical exam, discussing your findings with the patient, and writing a note. Cases that vary from this idealized format and how to approach them will be discussed separately in Chapter 6, Atypical Cases.

■ GETTING STARTED

The exam will begin when you are shown to your first station. You will be positioned in front of the door and be allowed to read a brief description of the patient and his or her reason for visiting.

Reading the Patient Description

The description will have the patient's name, age, gender, reason for the visit, vital signs, a description of the tasks that need to be completed, and possibly some other introductory information, depending on the case. You will be given time to read the information and compose yourself before entering the room. Your goal at this point in the case is to mentally compose your own checklists and prepare to meet your patient. The checklists you compose should be your best estimation of what the actual checklists will look like. Having an imaginary checklist will give structure to your visit.

Developing your Checklists

In a typical case there are two checklists that will be used to evaluate you. One for the history you take and another for the physical exam you perform. You need to be able to imagine what both checklists will be like for that case in the moments you have while reading the patient's introductory information. Your checklists need to be broad. For instance if the introductory information says that the patient has chest pain and you focus immediately on the heart, you may forget to consider a number of noncardiac sources of chest pain that will undoubtedly be on both checklists. The checklists you imagine are meant to serve as a guide for your patient interaction. You should try to come up with at least six items for each checklist to get you started. When considering the history checklist remember that there are only nine general causes of human disease, that follow the mnemonic VINDICATE:

1. Vascular
2. Infectious
3. Neoplastic
4. Degenerative
5. Immunologic
6. Congenital
7. Added (toxin/poison/drug)
8. Trauma
9. Electrolytes/metabolic

Use these general causes of disease to formulate a mental list of possible reasons for the patient's symptoms and a checklist of items that need to be discussed with the patient to compose a complete history.

When reading the patient introduction you should also consider the components of a physical exam that may apply to the case. When devising your physical exam checklist, focus on body regions and organ systems and not specific organs. This will also help keep you from being too focused right away. Major body regions, presented roughly from head to toe, are:

1. Head and neck
2. Chest
3. Abdomen
4. Pelvis
5. Extremities
6. Skin
7. Nerves
8. Psychiatric

You should know how to properly evaluate all organs in each body region. Thinking of the body by regions will prevent you from limiting your exam to one organ. For example, if a patient presents with chest pain it is easy to focus only on the heart. However, an ideal exam for chest pain should involve the entire chest, abdomen, and skin/body wall to evaluate for pulmonary, gastrointestinal, and external/traumatic causes of chest pain. For chest pain, it is probably not necessary to examine the other body regions listed. When you develop your physical exam checklist, be flexible as information you gather in the history may alter your physical exam somewhat.

■ MEETING YOUR PATIENT

Plan your introduction ahead of time so that you are comfortable with it. The nature of the exam will require you to think on your feet, and anything that you can make routine ahead of time will be one less source of potential surprise during the exam. Introducing yourself and getting started may be the most difficult parts of each case. Use the following plan for each patient:

1. Knock on the door (You must do this!)
2. Greet the patient *by name* while making eye contact (Hello Mr. Johnson)
3. Introduce yourself by name (My name is Dr. Julie Smith)
4. Ask the patient what is wrong (What brings you in today?)

Greet the patient warmly. Your opening lines will set the mood for the interview and play a big role in the patient's assessment of your interpersonal skills. If you begin with the above greeting and you have your checklists in mind you are on the road to success.

Before going further with your patient interaction you must consider the objectives for the case. Your evaluation will be based on the case objectives and it is critical that you understand what they are and adhere to them. For instance, suppose you have a patient complaining of pain with urination and the stated objective is to take a sexual history. It is critical that you actually take a sexual history and not get sidetracked taking a complete history or focusing on some other aspect of your patient. The checklist will only contain items that pertain to the stated objective. *You could have a flawless interaction with your patient, but if you miss the objective you will fail that case.* Understand your task exactly and proceed without distraction.

The following sections about history taking, performing a physical exam, communicating with your patients, and writing a medical note assume that you have a certain amount of experience with each of these components. The discussion is limited to how each component applies to the USMLE Step 2 CS. If you need more information about any of the following components, please refer to a basic textbook on proper history taking and physical exam techniques.

■ TAKING PATIENT HISTORIES

To effectively take a patient's medical history, determine exactly what you are trying to accomplish and stay focused. You may be asked to take a complete history on a patient or a focused history based on a patient's specific complaints. The components of a complete history are outlined below. You may perform only certain parts of the history for a given patient based on the specific situation and case objectives.

Chief Complaint

The chief compliant is usually one sentence or phrase that is a summary of the patient's problem. The chief complaint will probably be elicited when you greet the patient and ask why he or she is coming to see you. The chief complaint may be stated in the patient description, but you must ask the patient what is wrong and hear the chief complaint for yourself. It is a great way to start your interaction with the patient.

History of Present Illness

This is the next logical step in discussing your patient's problem. It provides details about the chief complaint such as how long the problem has existed or whether he or she has had the problem before. This is probably the most important part of the history, and you will have greater success with your questioning if you have an organized approach. Begin the history of present illness by using the alphabetical mnemonic PQRST.

P IS FOR PROVOKES

Ask the patient what provokes his or her symptoms, what makes the symptoms better, and what treatments, if any, have already been tried.

Q IS FOR QUALITY

Ask the patient to further define the quality of the symptoms. If the symptom is pain it can be dull, sharp, or achy. If the patient is coughing the cough can be dry, productive of sputum, or blood tinged.

R IS FOR RADIATION

Ask the patient exactly where on his or her body the symptoms exist, whether they affect any other body part, or if the location has changed since the onset.

S IS FOR SEVERITY

Ask the patient how bad the symptoms are. For pain you may ask the patient to rate it on a numeric scale. For other symptoms, such as shortness of breath, you may ask whether the symptoms limit physical activity or cause absence from work.

T IS FOR TIME

Ask your patient about the onset of symptoms, how long they last, and whether the symptoms come and go.

The above questioning is excellent for characterizing pain, which will probably be the chief complaint for many of your patients. The PQRST questions can better define practically any symptom. Use the PQRST questions for your initial questioning based on the chief complaint.

Earlier you were asked to recall the nine general causes of human disease (VINDICATE) to guide you in forming a differential diagnosis. After asking the PQRST questions you should consider VINDICATE again and use it to remember more specific questions for the history. Questioning your patient using PQRST followed by VINDICATE is an easy and organized way of developing a broad list of things to ask the patient. The lists are meant to help you remember categories of diseases and serve as a guide to the questions you actually ask. Do not take it too literally. For example, if your patient has chest pain and you are considering an infectious cause, do not ask, "Do you have an infection?" Instead you should ask more realistic questions that will tell you if the patient has an infection such as "Have you had a fever or chills?" You may then follow up with "Are any of your close contacts sick?" The lists, when used as a general guide, can serve as a springboard for practically all your questioning, and you will pick up a lot of checklist points using this organized approach. It may not be necessary to cover every item on the list for every patient, and your judgment will tell you what you can safely leave out. Using the PQRST questions to get you started and VINDICATE for the specifics will get you most of the history checklist points.

In many cases you will be asked to take a focused history based on a given patient problem, instead of a complete history. Often, the history of present illness by itself will provide a significant portion of the focused history with a few additions based on the case specifics.

Past Medical History

The past medical history is a list of the patient's prior diagnoses. Unless the patient's past medical history is somehow relevant to the current problem, the patient will probably say he or she has no past medical history when asked. Standardized patients must memorize their lines and it doesn't benefit anyone to have them recite a list of illnesses that are completely unrelated to the current problem. Therefore, if the patient does mention specific past medical problems you should pay attention because they are probably somehow related to the current problem.

Family History

The family history is designed to detect risk factors for a specific illness or help make a diagnosis based on the fact that some diseases tend to run in families. For cases that don't specifically mention a family history, reproductive problems, or genetics, asking one or two open-ended questions about the overall health of the patient's parents, siblings, and children is all that is necessary. More specifics may be needed if the case calls for it in some way. In general, the information that stands to be gained on the USMLE with an extensive family history is minimal and you should plan to be brief.

Social History

The social history can include a variety of things like the patient's living situation and employment that may be important for patients with a social or psychiatric problem. For common medical complaints, the social history can usually be reduced to a discussion about sexual practices and the use of tobacco, alcohol, and street drugs. *You must remember to ask every reproductive age female patient whether she could be pregnant.* It is an almost guaranteed checklist item and your entire interaction with the patient may be different based on the answer. In general, people like to talk about their lives, making the social history a potential time waster on the exam if it is not used properly. In most cases you should try to keep this part of the history short.

Medications

This part of the history is basically a list of medications the patient is taking. In reality these lists can be enormous, but for the exam the standardized patients must memorize their lines. Therefore, it is not practical for patients to recite a huge list of irrelevant medications. If you ask, patients will probably tell you they are not taking any medications, unless they are somehow related to the current problem. If the patient indicates that he or she is taking a medication, it is very likely to have a role in the case. You must ask the patient why he or she is using the medication if it is not obvious. Suspect the disease the medication is treating or side effects as having a role in the patient encounter. Whether you ask about medications is a common checklist item even if the patient isn't on any. Unless medication use is totally unrelated to the case objectives, plan to ask each patient if he or she is taking any medications.

Allergies

If you ask, most patients will probably tell you that they have no allergies unless an allergy has a specific role in the current case. Again, there is no reason for the standardized patient to memorize a list of allergies unless they matter somehow. Unless the patient's allergies are clearly not a part of your objectives for a case, plan to ask everyone if they have allergies. It too is a common checklist item.

Review of Systems

By the time you get this far in the history the patient has revealed information that should give you an idea of the diagnosis. The review of systems is a series of brief questions, often with yes or no answers, which help further define what you have already learned about the patient. The review of systems for a given organ system consists of any questions that will help you determine a diagnosis. Positive and negative findings are important in this setting, and both will be crucial later when you write your note and justify your differential diagnosis. Keep the review of systems brief and focused on the chief complaint.

The above items encompass a complete history. Some cases may require that you gather more information than others or have a different emphasis depending on the situation. If you think a specific question may be important, but unlikely to further the case, ask it anyway. Sometimes a specific question has little role in the case, but will be on the checklist as something you should have explored.

You will be allowed to take notes during your questioning just as you would during a real patient interview. Take a moment at the beginning of the interview and separate your paper into sections to keep you organized. In all cases you will have to write a note after your patient interaction. Staying organized from the beginning will save time and effort later. Also, make a note of the patient's name so you remember it during your interview and for the note you will write.

You must be specific with the questions you ask during the history. You want your style of questioning to match the expectations of the standardized patient and the checklists. If your questions are too vague you may think you covered something that the standardized patient won't give you credit for. For example, if you ask a patient whether a medical problem affects his or her life in any way, the question may be too vague. The checklist may have similar item on it, but it may be worded differently. The checklist may require that you ask whether the problem keeps the patient from working full time. Whether you get the check may be somewhat dependent on the standardized patient. To keep the scoring objective there are rather strict requirements regarding how close you need to be to a checklist item for it to count. In general, your question needs to have the exact meaning as the checklist question for you to get credit. Consider what information you are trying to gather and formulate the question as specifically as you can.

■ PERFORMING A PHYSICAL EXAM

As it is with the history, the key to a successful physical exam is knowing exactly what is expected of you and executing it without missing anything or performing a lot of extra tasks. *If you perform a flawless physical exam that was not required you will fail that case.* For the sake of time, most cases that require a physical exam will probably require only a focused physical exam pertaining to a specific system or body region. Remember as you approach the physical exam that the examiners specifically disallow some components of the physical exam. The USMLE instructions state that a rectal exam, pelvic exam, genitourinary exam, female breast exam, or corneal reflex exam is prohibited.[2] *For patients that need one of the prohibited exams, you should state the need for the specific exam to your patient and write it in your note as part of your plan.*

Earlier, you were asked to formulate your physical exam checklist by body region to keep you from thinking too specifically. In cases that require a history and physical exam, you will learn things during the history that allow you to focus your physical exam. In general, it is best to start with an organized plan for the physical exam with a focus on specific body regions. As you perform the exam, say out loud what you are doing and why you are doing it. For example,"I am now going to assess the size of your liver by feeling below your ribs." These statements will make your patients more comfortable, get them involved with the physical exam, and leave no doubt as to what portion of the exam you are performing for scoring purposes. When preparing to perform a physical exam, consider the following items:

What Needs to Be Examined?

In general, the answer will be one or more of the body regions listed earlier as dictated by the history you take and the case objectives. Remember to think broadly, as sometimes an organ that is distant from the site of the symptoms should be checked as part of a thorough exam. Think of the patient from head to toe to stay organized.

Components of the Physical Exam

In general, a complete physical exam for any body region includes observation, palpation, percussion, and auscultation. Clearly, some body parts will not require each one. For example, you would never use percussion on a patient's head. These are meant to be guidelines, and it should be obvious when you should leave something out. Consider the following tasks for each organ in the body region the patient is complaining about:

1. OBSERVATION
Your observation begins the moment you see the patient and ends when you leave the room. Your observation includes both the patient as a whole and the specific organ or body region you are examining. When considering the whole patient, observe his or her affect, mannerisms, clothing, smell, gait, and hygiene. You will learn a lot about the patient's mood, goals for the meeting, overall health, and ability to care for him- or herself. For specific organs or body regions, you should start the physical exam by observing the patient's body part of concern in it natural state. Of note, you cannot properly observe the patient if he or she is fully clothed. You must ask the patient to expose the area to be examined.

2. PALPATION
After observing, touch the area being examined and feel for any abnormalities. You must remember to wash your hands before and after you touch the patient. Gloves may be provided for you and you may use them if you like, but you should still wash your hands first. Start with light, superficial palpation and progress to deeper palpation. If the patient is in pain, be gentle and don't elicit the pain more than necessary. As a rule, most beginners are too soft with palpation. Don't be bashful. Patients come to the doctor and expect to be touched, and you cannot perform an adequate exam if you are too gentle.

3. PERCUSSION
Percussion can be performed in a variety of ways. The most effective way involves placing the middle finger of one hand flat on the patient's body and striking that finger with the middle finger of the other hand. Percussion

sounds are either dull, indicating an internal solid area or resonant, indicating a relatively hollow internal area. This technique is generally used during the pulmonary and abdominal exams.

4. AUSCULTATION

Auscultation involves listening first without the stethoscope if sounds are audible and then with the stethoscope. You may want to tell the patient what you are doing when you are listening without the stethoscope because it may not be obvious. You should be able to recognize and describe all the sounds that are associated with certain disease states, particularly for the heart and lungs. Don't forget to warm the stethoscope before placing it on the patient.

Examination Technique

Remember that the standardized patient is not only watching what you examine, but also your examination technique. You must be comfortable performing all the components of a basic physical exam. A complete review of the physical exam is beyond the scope of this book. You should have experience performing a physical exam, and if you are unsure of your technique, get a basic physical exam book and a partner and practice. Playing the role of the doctor and the patient will allow you to perform the exam and experience what the exam should feel like to the patient.

The Physical Exam

Be prepared to perform the following components of the physical exam:

GENERAL EXAM AND VITAL SIGNS

Observe the patient for any abnormalities in speech, gait, hygiene, dress, etc. Vital signs are posted in the introductory information on the door. You can recheck the vital signs, but you should only recheck them if they have a central role in the case, such as a patient presenting for a blood pressure check. Otherwise rechecking the vitals takes valuable time away from your patient encounter.

HEAD, EYES, EARS, NOSE, AND THROAT

You will not be allowed to use an ophthalmoscope, but you will be expected to use the otoscope for examining the ears, nose, and pharynx. Be prepared to examine the thyroid gland, lymph nodes, jugular veins, and carotid arteries for bruits.

CHEST

The chest examination includes both the heart and lungs. **You will have to perform this examination on multiple patients and it behooves you to have it down.** Be prepared to inspect, palpate, percuss, and auscultate your way through the chest exam. You should know the different heart sounds and breath sounds, how to describe them, and what they mean. *Shortness of breath and chest pain are among the most common exam topics.*

ABDOMINAL/PELVIC EXAM

Be prepared to inspect, palpate, percuss, and auscultate in each abdominal quadrant. Be aware of the organs you are examining and the technique used to examine them. *Abdominal pain is another favorite exam topic.* Rectal and pelvic exams are not allowed on the test. You will have patients that need these exams though, so you must know when they are necessary. When they are needed, say so in your note as part of the plan. The rectal exam, in general, is not performed as often as it should be because it is uncomfortable for everyone. It should be a part of any complete abdominal or pelvic exam, and if you are in doubt, include it.

SKIN

Always examine the skin in the area the patient is complaining about. The skin is one of the few organs that is readily visible. Having a patient with a skin finding that is covered by the gown is a great way for the examiners to test the thoroughness of your physical exam.

NEUROLOGICAL EXAM

Be able to test cranial nerves, motor function, sensation, cerebellar function, and reflexes.

PSYCHIATRIC

Be ready to give a screening mental status exam, interpret the findings, and explain them to the patient.

■ COMMUNICATING WITH YOUR PATIENT

While taking the history and performing the physical exam most of your verbal communication is organized into brief, specific questions. After the history and physical exam you will be expected to answer your patient's questions and discuss the treatment, prognosis, and follow-up. Many communication challenges, such as breaking bad news, are easier on the test because the patient is not real. Other things are more difficult because you may be nervous. Others yet are confusing because both you and your patient are acting and relying a great deal on falsified expressions, mood, and behavior. Regardless, your verbal and nonverbal communication skills will be closely assessed throughout the exam, and you will have cases specifically designed to test those skills. Your patient may ask you questions, but there are certain things (listed below) you must be prepared to offer without being asked. As always, having an organized approach will help you through this part of the exam. Before addressing your patient, consider again your objectives and make sure you are fulfilling them as you go through the following sequence:

Explain Your History and Physical Exam Findings

Keep this simple! All that is required here is a very basic description, and the use of medical jargon is specifically discouraged. For example, you may start your discussion by saying: "Given that you came to me with symptoms of abdominal pain, I examined your belly and found a tender area on the right."

Provide a Differential Diagnosis

The differential diagnosis that you tell the patient should include at least 3 things. Remember that you do not necessarily have to be right. The patient's checklist is more likely to require that you gave a differential than it is to require specific items. Many diagnoses are not made based on the history and physical exam alone, and you will not be expected to be exactly right. It is most important that you try, even if you don't know. For example you may try saying: "Given your physical exam findings, I think you may have an irritated gallbladder, but it may be a stomach ulcer, or an inflamed pancreas."

Discuss Your Plan

Here you should mention what further testing needs to be done if any, the treatment, and when the patient should plan to see you again. It is very important to include these items in your discussion with the patient. If you don't know the plan you should be very general ("I plan to order some tests to help me make a diagnosis") or guess. Again, the checklist is more likely to require that you made a general statement about the plan than it is to require specifics. It is best if you know the plan, but if it comes down to guessing or not mentioning it, it is better to make your best guess than to leave out the plan.

Discuss Your Prognosis

You must provide a general statement about how you expect the patient's problem to evolve. Once again, if you don't know, it is better to be general or guess than to have not covered this at all.

Have a Smooth Ending

You want to leave the patient with a good impression, as he or she will evaluate you moments after you leave the exam room. Plan to have a way to end each case that sounds professional and includes the patient's name. You may provide a brief summary of what you have discussed followed by a good closing such as "Thank you for coming today, Mr. Johnson. I will discuss our visit with a senior physician and get back to you."

Other Points

As you go through the above sequence there are several general effective communication techniques that will help you make a good impression on your patients.

REMEMBER YOUR MANNERS

When talking to your patient make eye contact, sit at the same level, use understandable words, look interested, and never interrupt your patient.

DON'T IGNORE A PATIENT'S QUESTION

In general it is expected that you provide the patient with information about his or her disease, the plan, and further treatment without being asked. Patients will sometimes ask questions, but they are not trying to help you or give you clues about what you should be discussing. If a patient asks a specific question it is probably for a reason. The question may lead to a dilemma, and its intent is to see that you respond and how you handle it. For example, you may have a patient with a sexually transmitted disease who asks you not to tell his or her sexual partner. In such cases it is important that you address the question and provide the best response you can. Do not let a difficult question or the lack of a good answer keep you from trying. Having the right answers in such cases is very difficult, and sometimes there may be no right answer. The fact that you don't ignore the question is more likely the point being tested than the actual answer you give.

TONE OF VOICE

When you are rushed or stressed as you may be on exam day it is easy to seem rude. It is particularly easy to become unpleasant if a patient is not cooperating with the interview. You may have a patient that is specifically trying to disrupt your interview by talking too much or continuously getting off the subject. Such a case may be testing your ability to stay calm and redirect the interview. Your tone of voice and the phrasing of your remarks are every bit as important as the actual words you are saying.

RESPOND TO YOUR PATIENT'S EMOTIONS

If a patient becomes emotional it is important that you acknowledge the emotion. ***Never plow through the objectives without considering the context of the interview.*** For example, you may have a patient presenting with difficulty sleeping who emotionally reveals the recent loss of a loved one during the interview. Your history objectives would be quite different for a grieving patient than they would be for a heavy coffee drinker. Pay attention to the situation and allow yourself to adapt if necessary.

PLAY ALONG

This book provides scripted lines designed to help you remember what to do in certain situations. You should use the scripts, but allow yourself to be flexible. If you are too rigid your responses will seem canned and insincere, which will detract from the effectiveness of your communication. This exam is a game of sorts and you can't be afraid to play along. This includes deviating from the script if necessary, and acting when the situation calls for it.

■ SPOKEN ENGLISH

If you are a native English speaker you can expect to pass this part of the exam. The assessment of your communication skills includes your grasp of spoken English. Everybody taking the Step 2 CS exam has probably passed Step 1 and Step 2 CK, and therefore probably has a solid understanding of written English. Reading and speaking, however, are quite different, and exams prior to the CS don't directly test your speaking skills. While it is not practical to learn an entire language in preparation for the USMLE Step 2 CS exam, there are certain things you can do to make the most of your skills and come across as an effective communicator.

Practice Speaking English

The most effective way to improve your English is by practicing. This basically involves using English at every opportunity, and pushing yourself to use new words. Occasionally ask someone who knows English well if there is anything you need to work on, like pronunciation. Many nonnative speakers develop habits and repeat the same mistakes time and again. Push yourself to improve.

Practice Speaking Medicine

Even for native speakers, learning medical jargon and medical abbreviations is not easy. You can anticipate encountering certain words and phrases in the medical field and on the exam. Give them special attention.

Listen for Understanding

This involves exposing yourself to English at every opportunity including other English speakers, television, radio, movies, or whatever means available. Force yourself to improve by paying attention to new words and looking them up if you are unsure of their meaning.

Practice Your Lines

This is probably the most effective way to get through the exam with as little work as possible. In the previous pages this book has outlined a number of phrases or questions that you can ask using the words exactly as they appear. While you cannot script everything you will say or hear on the exam, you can get a long way by practicing the lines you know you will say and making sure you are saying them correctly.

Take an English Course

Check with a local college or university and take an introductory course in English. Take the course well before the exam so that you have time to build on the skills you learn.

Live in an English-Speaking Country

While this may seem like rather unusual advice for exam preparation, if your goal is to practice medicine in the United States, you will eventually need to get some first-hand experiences. Immersion is the best way to learn the language and medical practices of physicians in the United States.

■ NOTE WRITING

When you finish with your patient all cases will require that you write a note. The note will be in template form with designated areas for the history, physical exam, differential diagnosis, and diagnostic work-up. You will have the option of writing the note on paper or typing the note on a keyboard. Unless you have excellent penmanship you should plan to type the note. A typed note will be easier for the evaluators to read and will make a better impression than a messy handwritten note. The notes need not be excessively long, but the better your typing skills, the more efficient you can be with your note. Additionally, certain common medical abbreviations are allowed in the note. You may be able to save some time by using them, but you should *not* make up any abbreviations, use nonstandard abbreviations, or use abbreviations that can confuse your meaning. The seconds you will save will not be worth the potential confusion. Also you do not necessarily have to use complete sentences, but remember this is a test of communication skills. The history is probably best written in complete sentences, while phrases are more appropriate for the physical exam part of the note. You will be allowed 10 minutes to write your note. You must remember to mention significant positive *and* negative findings of the history and physical exam. The typical note will require the following things:

Differential Diagnosis

Though it will not appear first on the note template, plan to start your note with the differential diagnosis. The rest of the note will come directly from it. You will need to list between two and five different diagnoses that may account for the patient's symptoms. Start with items that are very likely to be the diagnosis and end with less likely possibilities. It is probably better to list as close to five items as possible, even if the last few are unlikely. In some cases you may have some evidence from the history or physical exam that doesn't completely support a particular diagnosis. That should not necessarily prevent you from putting it on your list. Symptoms and exam findings for a given illness vary, and your list will be very short if you exclude things too easily. It is okay if you end up with a list of one or two strong possibilities followed by others that don't fit as well.

History

You will be asked to describe the pertinent positive and negative findings from each of the various components of the history (present illness, past medical, social, family, and review of systems). Once again the key to success is understanding exactly what is expected of you. A complete recap of your interview is not feasible and your note is going to be limited by time. Think again about PQRST and VINDICATE. You want to state all of the positive findings that these questions produced, and list the negative findings (often obtained in the review of systems) that are pertinent to the differential diagnosis. Consider your differential diagnosis as an argument that needs support from the rest of your note. Imagine that you have to convince someone that your differential diagnosis is correct. You need to have positive and negative findings from the history that strongly support the first few items on the list. You will probably have less convincing evidence for the last few items. If you don't have any positive or negative evidence for an item on your differential diagnosis, you may want to rethink your differential diagnosis. If an item in your history has no relevance to the differential, you do not need to include it in your note.

In reality, most medical notes are full of abbreviations and incomplete sentences. Because of the exam's emphasis on communication you should plan to use complete sentences and minimize abbreviations for the history as much as time will allow. Also, pay attention to spelling. Begin the history part of the note with: "The patient is a ___-year-old male or female who presents with . . ."

Physical Exam

For the physical exam part of the note you will be asked to discuss the pertinent positive and negative findings relating to the patient's chief complaint. Again, you should use your differential diagnosis as a guide, and pretend it is an argument that needs supporting evidence. The important positive and negative physical exam findings are those that strengthen your differential diagnosis. If you don't have positive and negative physical exam evidence for a particular diagnosis, you may want to rethink the diagnosis. The typical report on a physical exam tends to have even more abbreviations than the history and usually is written in list format without complete sentences. Despite the exam's emphasis on communication and proper use of English, you may use well-known abbreviations and phrases on this part of the note to save time. As a rule, you should not describe your physical exam findings using the word normal. The graders do not know if you know what normal is. Describe your findings instead, even if the description is that of a normal healthy organ system.

Diagnostic Workup

You will be asked to list up to five items that would be immediately necessary for a final diagnosis. **Beware: these items are strictly for the diagnosis and should not include treatments.** Your diagnostic workup should also be derived from the differential diagnosis. Start with the first items on your differential and consider what tests would be necessary to confirm your suspicion. In general, order a lab test if there is one available for the diagnosis you are considering and a radiographic study if there is a reason to visualize the affected organs. You can only list up to five items, so start with the first (most important) items on your differential. Common important initial tests are an ECG, complete blood count, basic chemistry, and some sort of visualization study such as an x-ray, ultrasound, or endoscopy, depending on the case. In this part of the note you should list any disallowed physical exam maneuvers (breast exam, rectal exam) if you think they are necessary. If you cannot relate a particular test to an item on the differential don't order the test.

■ SUMMARY OF THE TYPICAL CASE

You will have better success on the exam if you have a plan with each of your patients. A plan for the typical case requiring a history, focused physical exam, discussion, and note has been presented and is summarized below. Remember that this is a general, idealized plan. Certain cases may require you to stray from the plan and you should be able to recognize when it is appropriate to do so.

- Read the case description and understand the objectives.
- Formulate your own history checklist using VINDICATE.
- Formulate your own physical exam checklist remembering the following body regions/organ systems: head and neck, chest, abdomen, pelvis, extremities, skin, nerves, psychiatric.
- Meet your patient: knock on the door, greet the patient by name while making eye contact, introduce yourself by name, and ask the patient what is wrong.
- Take the history including the chief complaint, the history of present illness including PQRST and VINDICATE, the past medical history, family history, social history, medications, and allergies, and review of systems.

- Make organized notes for yourself for later when you have to write your note.

- Perform a focused physical exam by observing, palpating, percussing, and auscultating the appropriate body regions.

- Explain your history and physical exam findings, provide a differential diagnosis, discuss the plan, follow-up, and prognosis.

- Write your note beginning with the differential diagnosis. View the differential diagnosis as an argument and the history and physical exam as supporting evidence designed to convince the reader you are correct.

6

Atypical Cases

Much of the book has been devoted to cases that follow the typical pattern of taking the history, performing the physical exam, communicating with the patient, and then writing the note. Indeed, most of your cases will adhere to this general pattern, but you may have encounters with a different format. You may have cases with more of a social or psychiatric theme. Some cases may not require a physical exam, but instead require that you talk to the patient at length. For example, you may be required to console a patient about a specific problem, deliver bad news about a patient's health, provide an interpretation of a test, or function in any number of common patient–doctor interactions. In these cases it is particularly important that you understand your objectives and adhere to them.

The following section discusses possible case formats that could be part of your exam. While you will not likely encounter all of these types of cases on your exam, they might be present on some of the exams.

■ THE PATIENT WITH A SECRET

You may have a patient with a newly positive pregnancy test, a newly diagnosed sexually transmitted disease, or a patient who has been physically or sexually abused. The patient will ask you not to tell his or her sexual partner, significant other, or parents and it will be up to you to know the rules and how to respond. Make it your goal to convince the patient to inform the necessary person or people of the problem. You may offer to be present, but avoid making threats about reporting the condition yourself, even if it is your legal obligation. Keep your bond with the patient. Most people can be made to see the necessity of doing what is right.

■ BEARING BAD NEWS

This type of station will require you to discuss a new diagnosis of a terminal disease such as cancer or HIV. If the patient doesn't know the diagnosis yet, you will need to break the news, discuss the details of the disease, and answer questions. Set the stage by providing a warning shot: "Mr. Johnson I'm afraid I have some bad news for you." Then give the news. Be prepared to discuss the disease, particularly the prognosis, treatment, and how it will affect his or her life. Ask about the patient's thoughts and feelings and social support system. Leave the patient by asking if there are any further questions and indicate that you can be reached if they have any questions later.

■ GET CONSENT

You may be required to get consent from a patient for a specific procedure or test. You must clearly explain what will be done, why it must be done, and the benefits, risks, and alternatives. You should explain what the test will feel like and what if anything will be done to minimize pain, bleeding, infection, etc. Explain the possible results and how they will alter the patient's care. Emphasize that the test or procedure is going to benefit him or her. If the patient declines to have the test or procedure, be accepting and find out why without being pushy or condescending.

■ FORGO TREATMENT

You may have a case of a patient needing a vital procedure or treatment who refuses care. Common examples include surgery, chemotherapy, and blood product administration. Ensure that the patient understands the consequences of refusal and that he or she is mentally capable of making the decision. Discuss the reasons for refusal and alternative treatments or procedures if there are any.

■ NONCOMPLIANT PATIENT

This type of case will involve a patient with a treatable illness that doesn't seem to want treatment or understand the need for treatment. It is important that you discuss the illness with the patient and the benefits of treatment. Ask if there is a particular reason that he or she is not using the treatment and consider a new treatment if it is somehow better suited. Your choice of words will be very important. Be careful not to scold or sound condescending.

■ PSYCHIATRIC PATIENT/MENTAL STATUS CHANGES

These cases will usually involve an elderly parent who is brought in by the son or daughter because of irregular behavior or somnolence. Depending on the situation, a medical cause for the altered behavior should be sought, and therefore the differential diagnosis and questioning using PQRST and VINDICATE apply. Your physical exam may be somewhat limited for psychiatric patients, but thorough chest and nerve examinations are probably necessary. You must also be prepared to perform a mental status examination and explain your findings. Any case involving someone other than you and the patient, such as a patient's family member, deserves special attention. *Be certain the patient is okay having the other person present during your interaction.* You should start your interview by asking to talk to the patient privately and then asking the patient in private if it is okay for others to join you. If there is someone in the room with the patient, your asking to see the patient privately is an almost guaranteed checklist item.

■ TOBACCO/ALCOHOL ADDICTION

First, explore whether the patient is interested in quitting. Your approach will be much different depending on the answer. The risks of continued use and the benefits of quitting should be emphasized to patients who aren't interested in quitting. Ask about prior attempts at quitting and the methods used. Assess the level of use (how often/how much). For alcohol remember the CAGE questions (need to Cut down, Annoyed by criticism, Guilt about using, Eye opener in the morning) for assessing dependence. Explain that you understand how difficult it is to quit. Provide encouragement and offer a specific plan (the patch or nicotine gum for smoking and hospitalization and support groups for alcoholism).

■ SUICIDAL PATIENT

You may have an acutely suicidal patient. It is most important that you assess the severity of the situation. Ask if the patient currently has a plan and whether he or she has access to a gun. You want to ask about prior suicide attempts and whether he or she has any thoughts of harming other people. Ask the patient why he or she doesn't want to live and try to discourage further suicidal thoughts. Explain the treatment options including hospital admission and counseling.

■ FAMILY COUNSELING

You may have a case where a couple with a personal or family history of an inheritable disease wants to have a baby. They will want to discuss the risk of passing the disease on to their child. You should be able to explain the mode of inheritance and the chance of their child having the disease based on the information the parents give you about themselves. Sickle cell anemia and other common genetic diseases with straightforward inheritance patterns are favorites in this setting.

■ THE HIDDEN FINDING

Some cases will have a clear set of objectives and appear very much like the typical case described earlier. Then you will see the patient and uncover a completely unsuspected finding that significantly alters the case objectives. For example, you may have a patient with a routine medical complaint on whom you discover severe belt lashings. You may have a patient who denies any past surgical history on whom you discover a surgical scar. The hidden finding will never be excessively difficult to find and you should not go looking for something in every case. Instead, the finding will be obvious if you are asking the right questions and performing the physical exam correctly. These cases are testing your thoroughness and ability to adapt during your interaction.

■ INTERPRETING A TEST

This type of station will provide a common medical test result and require that you explain the results to a patient or write a note explaining the findings. Common examples include an ECG, chest x-ray, or routine lab data like a complete blood count or basic chemistry. In general, the results will not be unusual and the interpretation not overly difficult. You should be ready to discuss the results, what they mean, and the plan for the patient.

7 Style and Grace

Because of the nature of the exam you can only prepare to an extent, and the rest depends on your patients, the cases you get, and how much experience you have with a given case topic. You must be able to improvise, and there are a variety of ways you can get caught off guard during a case. The following is a list of commonly occurring mishaps and how you can be prepared for them and recover with style and grace.

■ THE UNCOMFORTABLE SILENCE

You may find yourself staring at a standardized patient with nothing to say. The best way to get around uncomfortable silences is to allow yourself to become comfortable with a slow-paced interview. It is not necessary to fill the entire time with questions and discussion. You can get a lot of information from a patient's body language and nonverbal cues. Your patient is expecting some silent time and you should not necessarily feel compelled to fill it. You should also have a line ready to jump-start things if you become haunted by the silence or feel that the interview is not progressing. Ask the patient "Is there anything else you think I should know about your problem?" or say "Please tell me more about that."

■ THE UNANSWERABLE QUESTION

You need to recognize which questions should have answers and which ones may not. In many cases if you don't know the answer it is okay to just say so. For example, some patients may have difficult questions about how long they will live or how bad their disease is. It may be okay to be rather vague or say that you are not sure. Alternatively, a patient with a specific medical problem may ask you about your treatment plan and you should definitely have an answer. When you sense that you are being asked a question that you should have an answer to and you don't, make up an answer. The standardized patients often will not know you are wrong or it may not matter to them if you are wrong. For example, a checklist item may require that you discussed medication side effects with the patient. It will probably not list all the side effects though, and the patient may not even know what they are. What matters is that you considered the side effects and gave some advice, not anything more specific. Obviously, it is best to know the answer, but if you don't you should not let the fear of being wrong keep you from answering. Guess and sound confident! It will probably earn you a checkmark, while saying nothing surely will not.

THE FEELING YOU SHOULD BE DOING MORE

You may be with a patient and find yourself completely unable to remember what you should do next. If this occurs you must remember the cues presented earlier. They provide a logical, organized approach to each case that is specifically designed to help you remember the next step. Ask the patient in a general way to tell you more about his or her problem to buy you some time to think about what your next step should be. Alternatively, you can ask the patient to give you a moment to think about what he or she is telling you as you remember your plan. Silence is okay, and it will create the feeling that you are not rushed. Each case will vary, but you should be spending most of the allotted time with each patient. If you are always the first examinee out in the hall at the end of each case, you may want to reconsider your lists and spend a little more time with each patient.

DISTRACTED BY REALITY

Your interaction with every patient will consist almost entirely of simulated feelings, discussion, and sometimes complex emotions. You may find yourself completely unable to get in the spirit of acting with some patients, and some standardized patients' attempts to simulate pain, emotion, or other symptoms may be downright humorous. You can get into big trouble quickly if you become removed from the acting and view the patient from the perspective of reality. If this happens to you, you should never let it show. You should never ask the patient how you are doing or make a remark about the checklist, scoring, or anything that will break the simulation. All of the checklist items require that you play along. During the exam, pretend your patients are family members and that you are sharing in their problems. Stay focused and be ready to play your role.

THE RAMBLING PATIENT

You need to be conscious of time during your patient encounters and you may have patients who want to talk about irrelevant things and lead you away from your task. In fact, there may be cases where a standardized patient is specifically instructed to talk too much to see how you handle it. Have a polite way of redirecting the patient and staying in control of the interview. Try saying, "I would like to help you with your problem. Let's talk more about it." Do not worry excessively about being rude in these settings. You must stay on task. It is better to politely interrupt a patient and complete the objectives than it is to be nice and let the patient waste all your time.

WHEN IN DOUBT

You may wonder if a particular part of the history or physical exam is necessary. The checklists are completed based on the questions you asked or the parts of the physical exam you performed. If you did something extra that was not on the checklist, you probably won't be penalized. If you forget something that is on the list, it will surely cost you. When in doubt, more is better as long as time allows. However, a shotgun approach will probably take from your rapport with the patient and your overall presentation. The nature of the checklist scoring method gives you credit for items accomplished but does not take points away for doing extra, irrelevant tasks. It is therefore probably wise to err on the side of doing more with your patients, not less. However, you must remain conscious of time and stay as focused as possible.

CHANGING THE SEQUENCE

The ideal patient encounter is often presented in the following sequence: taking a history, performing a physical exam, discussing the findings, and writing the note occurring in that order. In reality you may think of questions later in the interview that should have been asked already, or you may remember to examine a particular organ after you have completed the exam. The above sequence is merely a guideline and you should *not* be afraid to go back and ask a question or perform a maneuver after you have moved on in your sequence of tasks. It is much better to take a thorough history and perform a proper physical exam that is somewhat disordered than it is to leave things out to maintain continuity.

8

Scoring

To achieve the best score you must understand exactly what is required of you on the exam.

■ EVALUATION CRITERIA

Remember that the exam is called the USMLE Step 2 Clinical Skills, and your clinical skills are exactly what are being tested. Your skill level is being assessed in 3 areas:

1. The history, physical exam, and patient note writing
2. Communication and interpersonal skills
3. Spoken English proficiency

Each of these items has been discussed in detail. It is equally important to realize what is not being tested. ***This is not a test of medical knowledge.*** While a certain amount of medical knowledge is required, it is not an integral part of scoring this exam, and you can expect the medical problems you encounter to be rather straightforward. Your patient interactions are being tested, and you should not let a lack of medical knowledge or factual tidbits keep you from having a fluid patient interaction. For the exam, be very general or guess at the facts if you don't know them.

Realize that your patient encounters are not complete patient encounters. ***You are being tested on your ability to establish rapport and effectively communicate as you take a history, perform an appropriate exam, develop a differential diagnosis, order initial tests, and document your encounter.*** Your encounter ends without test results, treatments, a plan for follow up, or many of the other difficult aspects of real patient care that may make this exam seem more involved than it is. The nature of the test requires that you leave your patient hanging to an extent. Realizing this before the exam will help you focus and keep your goals attainable.

It is also important to realize that most USMLE Step 2 CS test takers are not yet physicians. The exam is intended to measure your ability to perform the objectives as a medical student in a supervised setting. You are not a finished product and your ability to follow the first several steps of a patient encounter is not required to be either. With that background, you must understand how you are evaluated.

■ EVALUATION METHOD

Your final evaluation is a grade of pass or fail. You must pass on all three evaluation criteria to get an overall pass. The best method of evaluation is one that provides an accurate indication of the competence of the examinee. The first exams using patient simulators used a general method of evaluation where examinees were observed and given a pass or fail rating based on the overall assessment of an experienced onlooker.[4] This method was rather subjective and checklists were introduced to improve scoring reliability. For the checklists to be functional and provide an accurate assessment they must contain items that are easily identified by the rater. The first checklists were developed that contained easily assessable items that weren't necessarily critical components of the case. For example, in a case of shortness of breath, it is much easier to tell if an examinee listened to the lungs than it is to tell if the examinee considered the severity of the symptoms and the imminence of respiratory failure. Because it is a more definable task, listening to the lungs would make the checklist, while the equally important critical assessment of the patient's breathing may not. This led to the checklists containing only easily identifiable tasks and provided an inaccurate assessment of examinees. Both the general, overall assessment and the checklists were improved and made to be as valid and reliable as possible. Some experts believe that the best method of assessment is a combination using both the general rating and checklist methods.[4] The USMLE Step 2 CS uses a combination of the methods.[2] The checklist is rather objective and it is completed based on whether the examinee performed certain easily assessable tasks. The overall rating is more subjective and it is based on estimations of how a minimally competent student would perform.

■ DETERMINING PASS AND FAIL

There are numerous methods of identifying a passing score and countless variables that determine which one is best. The best scoring method for a clinical test must provide a true measure of competence. The method must balance the risks of passing incompetent students with the problem of remediating excessive failures. It must also consider the meaning of the particular exam. For example, the consequence of failing a medical school clerkship exam is much different from failing a licensing exam and being barred from a particular career. What represents a fair passing cut point should be different in these settings.[5] The Angoff and borderline methods of standard setting have emerged as accurate and rational for clinical exams such as the USMLE Step 2 CS.[6] The Angoff method involves a group of experienced medical educators who independently estimate how many checkmarks a marginal student would get on a given checklist. The results are discussed as a group, and a passing number of checkmarks is determined after working out any disagreements. The borderline method requires experienced educators to fill out a checklist during an exam and then provide an overall rating of excellent, good, borderline, or fail for the student. The avenge number of checkmarks obtained by those students ranked overall as borderline becomes the minimum number needed to pass. The minimum passing score for the USMLE Step 2 CS is probably determined using one of these methods.

Practice Cases

The remaining pages contain several practice cases. Each case begins with a brief description of the patient and your objectives for the visit. The descriptions are similar to what you will learn about your patients prior to seeing them on the exam. After reading the patient information you should formulate your own checklists for the history and physical exam.

Develop your checklists using the strategy presented in Chapter 5, Seeing Your Patients. Consider PQRST and VINDICATE for the history checklist and body regions with observation, palpation, percussion, and auscultation for the physical exam checklist. You should use this thought process and consider every step for each case. Be aware that some questions in the history could fit into more than one place. For example, asking a patient if he or she has ever had a sexually transmitted disease could fall under the infectious part of VINDICATE in the history of present illness, the past medical history, or the social history. Remember to be flexible with your history taking. As long as you remember to ask the question, it is not important to have it rigidly categorized. Additionally, many of the steps will not apply to each case. If you think a particular question or physical exam maneuver would be irrelevant or inappropriate in a given setting, skip it and move on. Cases will almost never require you to ask everything from PQRST and VINDICATE.

A completed checklist with simulated patient answers is provided in each case for comparison. After developing your checklists you should practice note writing based on the history checklist questions and answers and the physical exam findings. A completed note from each case is provided at the end of this chapter for comparison. Completing the practice cases will get you used to using an organized approach to your cases.

CASE 1

Mr. John Davis is a 47-year-old male who has come to your office because of a persistent cough.

Vital signs:

Temperature: 100.1°F $(37.8°C)$
Blood pressure: 124/82 mmHg
Pulse: 68
Respirations: 14

Mr. Davis is the director of a local homeless shelter and upon meeting him, you see that he is thin and coughs frequently. He is not having difficulty breathing. You have 15 minutes to take a history and perform a focused physical exam on Mr. Davis.

PREDICTED CHECKLIST

History Checklist:

_____
_____
_____
_____
_____
_____
_____
_____

Physical Exam Checklist:

_____
_____
_____
_____
_____
_____
_____

CASE 1 (continued)

SAMPLE CHECKLIST

History Checklist:

PQRST

P is for **Provokes**:

    ✓ Asked if anything makes the cough worse (Physical activity)

    ✓ Asked if I had tried treating the cough (Yes, cold medicine doesn't help)

Q is for **Quality**:

    ✓ Asked if the cough was dry, productive of sputum, or bloody (Cough is productive and sputum is often blood tinged)

R is for **Radiation**: Not applicable

S is for **Severity**:

    ✓ Asked if I feel short of breath (No)

    ✓ Asked if cough limits my daily activities or keeps me awake (Yes, it keeps me awake)

T is for **Time**:

    ✓ Asked how long I had the cough (1 month)

VINDICATE

Vascular:

    ✓ Asked if I am immobile for long periods of time (No)

    ✓ Asked if I have ever had a blood clot (No)

Infectious:

    ✓ Asked if I have had a fever or chills (Yes, my temperature has been about 100°F)

    ✓ Asked I if I have had night sweats (Yes, the sheets are all wet when I wake up)

    ✓ Asked about prior tuberculosis exposure (Often, many shelter residents have tuberculosis)

    ✓ Asked about last PPD test (1 year ago, it was negative)

Neoplastic:

    ✓ Asked if I have lost weight (Yes, 10 pounds in the last month)

Degenerative: Not applicable

Immunologic: Not applicable

Congenital: Not applicable

(**A**dded) Toxin/poison/drugs:

    ✓ Asked if I smoke (No, never have)

    ✓ Asked about exposure to hazardous material like asbestos or silica (No)

CASE 1 (continued)

Trauma: Not applicable

Electrolytes/metabolic: Not applicable

Other history:

Past medical history, family history, social history, medications, and allergies: Noncontributory

Review of systems: Has fatigue and weight loss. No headache, sore throat, chest pain, shortness of breath, nausea, vomiting, constipation, diarrhea, malaise, or lethargy.

Physical Exam Checklist:

    ✓ Washed hands before the exam
    ✓ Asked to untie gown

Head and neck:

    ✓ Palpated for enlarged lymph nodes (None palpable)

Chest:

    ✓ Observed chest wall for symmetric expansion/contraction (Symmetric expansion and contraction)
    ✓ Percussed on my back (Resonant percussion in all fields)
    ✓ Listened to my lungs in more than 4 places in the front and back (Lungs clear to auscultation)
    ✓ Listened to heart in more than 3 places (Regular rate and rhythm)

Abdomen: Not applicable

Pelvis: Not applicable

Extremities:

    ✓ Checked fingertips for clubbing (No clubbing)

Skin:

    ✓ Checked skin over chest (No lesions or scars)

Nerves: Not applicable

Psychiatric: Not applicable

You should have gotten at least 17 of the 24 possible checkmarks.

CASE 1 (continued)

YOUR NOTE

Differential Diagnosis (list up to 5 in order of likelihood)

1.

2.

3.

4.

5.

History (including positives and negatives from history of present illness, past medical history, family history, social history, and review of systems)

_____

_____

_____

_____

_____

_____

Physical Exam (consisting of positives and negatives relevant to the chief complaint)

_____

_____

_____

_____

_____

_____

Diagnostic Workup (up to 5 items necessary for further diagnosis)

1.

2.

3.

4.

5.

(see p. 121 for sample note)

CASE 2

Ms. Paula Smith is a 27-year-old female who has come to see you for diarrhea and abdominal cramping. She has not had an appetite and she has lost 7 pounds since the symptoms started.

Vital signs:

Temperature: 100.0°F $(37.7°C)$
Blood pressure: 118/76 mmHg
Pulse: 70
Respirations: 14

Upon meeting Ms. Smith you see that she is an ill-appearing female in no acute distress. You have 15 minutes to take a history and perform a focused physical exam on Ms. Smith.

PREDICTED CHECKLIST

History Checklist:

_____
_____
_____
_____
_____
_____
_____
_____

Physical Exam Checklist:

_____
_____
_____
_____
_____
_____
_____

CASE 2 (continued)

SAMPLE CHECKLIST

History Checklist:

PQRST

P is for **Provokes**:

    __✓__ Asked if anything makes the diarrhea/cramping worse (Meals)

    __✓__ Asked if I had tried treating the diarrhea (Yes, Imodium/Loperamide provides temporary relief, but it always comes back)

Q is for **Quality**:

    __✓__ Asked if stool is watery, formed, or bloody (Stool is watery and never bloody)

    ____ Asked if stool is black or particularly foul smelling (Stool is watery and brown with no particularly bad odor)

R is for **Radiation**: Not applicable

S is for **Severity**:

    __✓__ Asked if I am fatigued (Yes, I haven't been eating and I have no energy)

    __✓__ Asked if the diarrhea/cramps have caused me to miss work, kept me awake, or kept me from daily activities (Yes, it keeps me up at night)

T is for **Time**:

    __✓__ Asked how long I have had the diarrhea (3 days)

    __✓__ Asked how often I have diarrhea (About 8 times per day)

VINDICATE

Vascular: Not applicable

Infectious:

    __✓__ Asked if I have had a fever or chills (Yes, my temperature has been about 100°F)

    __✓__ Asked if I have been camping or traveled anywhere recently (No)

    __✓__ Asked if I have eaten raw fish or unpasteurized dairy products (No)

    __✓__ Asked about recent antibiotic use (No)

    __✓__ Asked about sick contacts (Yes, I work at a daycare and many of the children are sick with diarrhea)

Neoplastic: Not applicable

Degenerative: Not applicable

Immunologic:

    __✓__ Asked if symptoms are worse when eating wheat or rye products (No)

Congenital: Not applicable

CASE 2 (continued)

(**A**dded) Toxin/poison/drugs:

_____Asked if I eat things that aren't considered food (No)
_____Asked if I use diet drinks or food with sorbitol (No)

Trauma: Not applicable

Electrolytes/metabolic:

_√__Asked if I am lactose intolerant or if symptoms are worse with dairy
products (No)
_√__Asked if I have thyroid disease (No)

Other history:

Past medical history, family history, and allergies: Noncontributory

Social history:

____Asked if I could be pregnant (No, not sexually active)

Medication:

_√_Asked if I take laxatives (No)

Review of systems: Has nausea and fatigue. No headache, sore throat, chest
pain, shortness of breath, or vomiting.

Physical Exam Checklist:

_√__Washed hands before the exam
_√__Asked to untie gown

Head and neck:

____Palpated thyroid gland (Normal size and contours)

Chest: Not applicable

Abdomen:

_√__Observed abdomen for distention (Mild distention)
_√__Palpated lightly and deeply in all quadrants (Diffuse tenderness with
deep palpation, normal sized liver and spleen, no masses)
_√__Percussed abdomen in all quadrants (Resonant throughout)
_√__Listened to abdomen in all quadrants (Hyperactive bowel sounds)

Pelvis: Not applicable

Extremities: Not applicable

Skin:

_√_Checked skin over abdomen (No lesions or scars)

Nerves: Not applicable

Psychiatric: Not applicable

You should have gotten at least 20 of the 28 possible checkmarks.

CASE 2 (continued)

YOUR NOTE

Differential Diagnosis (list up to 5 in order of likelihood)

1.

2.

3.

4.

5.

History (including positives and negatives from history of present illness, past medical history, family history, social history, and review of systems)

_____

_____

_____

_____

_____

_____

Physical Exam (consisting of positives and negatives relevant to the chief complaint)

_____

_____

_____

_____

_____

_____

Diagnostic Workup (up to 5 items necessary for further diagnosis)

1.

2.

3.

4.

5.

(see p. 122 for sample note)

CASE 3

Susan Anderson is a 26-year-old female graduate student who has made an urgent appointment to see you for abdominal pain.

Vital signs:

Temperature: 99.9°F 37,7
Blood pressure: 120/77 mmHg
Pulse: 74
Respirations: 16

Upon meeting Ms. Anderson, you see that she is lying flat and motionless on the examination table. You have 15 minutes to take a history and perform a focused physical exam on Ms. Anderson.

PREDICTED CHECKLIST

History Checklist:

_____

_____

_____

_____

_____

_____

_____

Physical Exam Checklist:

_____

_____

_____

_____

_____

_____

_____

CASE 3 (continued)

SAMPLE CHECKLIST

History Checklist:

PQRST

P is for **Provokes**:

___✓ Asked if anything makes the pain worse (Movement)
___✓ Asked if I had tried treating the pain (No)

Q is for **Quality**:

___✓ Asked if pain is dull, sharp, or achy (Pain is sharp)

R is for **Radiation**:

___✓ Asked if the pain radiates anywhere (It started in the middle of my abdomen and is now on the lower right side)

S is for **Severity**:

___ Asked me to rate the pain on a scale of 1–10, 10 being the worst (The pain is 7/10)

T is for **Time**:

___✓ Asked when the pain started (After lunch about 10 hours ago. I haven't eaten since)

VINDICATE

Vascular: Not applicable

Infectious:

___✓ Asked if I have diarrhea (No)
___✓ Asked if I have had a fever or chills (No)

Neoplastic: Not applicable

Degenerative: Not applicable

Immunologic: Not applicable

Congenital: Not applicable

(**A**dded) Toxin/poison/drugs: Not applicable

Trauma: Not applicable

Electrolytes/metabolic:

___ Asked when I last had a bowel movement (2 days ago and it was normal)
___✓ Asked about blood in the urine and whether I have had kidney stones (No, neither)
___ Asked about last menstrual period (2 weeks ago and regular)

CASE 3 (continued)

Other history:

Past medical history

____√____Asked if I have had my appendix removed or other abdominal
surgery (No)

Family history and allergies: Noncontributory

Social history:

____√____Asked if I could be pregnant (No, I am not sexually active)
____√____Asked about previous sexually transmitted diseases (No previous
sexually transmitted diseases)

Review of systems: Has nausea, loss of appetite, and vomited once. No night
sweats, weight loss, headaches, sore throat, chest pain, shortness of breath,
urinary pain/frequency, vaginal discharge, diarrhea, constipation, malaise,
or lethargy.

Physical Exam Checklist:

____√____Washed hands before the exam
____√____Asked to untie gown

Head and neck: Not applicable

Chest: Not applicable

Abdomen:

____√____Observed abdomen for distention (There is mild distention)
____√____Palpated lightly and deeply in all quadrants (Profound lower right
tenderness with light palpation, significant rebound tenderness
and muscular resistance to the exam, normal sized liver and spleen,
no masses)
____√____Percussed on abdomen (Resonant throughout)
____√____Percussed firmly over both kidneys (No tenderness)
____√____Listened to abdomen in all quadrants (Hypoactive bowel sounds)

Pelvis: Exam deferred

Extremities:

____√____Asked me to lay on my left side and extended my right leg at the
hip (No pain)
____√____Asked me to lay on my back and rotated my right leg at the hip
(Pain is elicited)

Skin:

____√____Checked skin over abdomen (No lesions or surgical scars)

Nerves: Not applicable

Psychiatric: Not applicable

You should have gotten at least 17 of the 24 possible checkmarks.

CASE 3 (continued)

YOUR NOTE

Differential Diagnosis (list up to 5 in order of likelihood)

1.

2.

3.

4.

5.

History (including positives and negatives from history of present illness, past medical history, family history, social history, and review of systems)

_____

_____

_____

_____

_____

_____

Physical Exam (consisting of positives and negatives relevant to the chief complaint)

_____

_____

_____

_____

_____

_____

Diagnostic Workup (up to 5 items necessary for further diagnosis)

1.

2.

3.

4.

5.

(see p. 123 for sample note)

CASE 4

Mr. Steve Clark is a 64-year-old male who has come to see you urgently for chest pain.

Vital signs:

Temperature: 98.4°F
Blood pressure: 150/92 mmHg
Pulse: 88
Respirations: 14

Upon meeting Mr. Clark you see that he is moderately overweight, diaphoretic, and appears troubled. He says he first noticed the pain when he was mowing the lawn. You have 15 minutes to take a history and perform a focused physical exam on Mr. Clark.

PREDICTED CHECKLIST

History Checklist:

_____
_____
_____
_____
_____
_____
_____
_____

Physical Exam Checklist:

_____
_____
_____
_____
_____
_____
_____
_____

CASE 4 (continued)

SAMPLE CHECKLIST

History Checklist:

PQRST

P is for **Provokes**:

    ✓ Asked if anything makes the pain worse (Physical activity. The pain occurred while I was mowing the lawn)

    ✓ Asked if I had tried treating the pain (Yes, I took aspirin but it didn't help)

Q is for **Quality**:

    ✓ Asked if pain is sharp, dull, crushing, or achy (The pain is burning and crushing)

R is for **Radiation**:

    ✓ Asked where the pain is (Under my sternum, in the middle of my chest)

    ✓ Asked if the pain radiates anywhere (Yes, the pain is also present in my neck and jaw)

S is for **Severity**:

    ✓ Asked me to rate the pain on a scale of 1–10, 10 being the worst (The pain is 8/10)

T is for **Time**:

    ✓ Asked how long I have had the pain (About 4 hours)

    ✓ Asked if I have had the pain before (Yes, I have had chest pain with activity before, but it always goes away with rest)

    ✓ Asked if I am still having the pain (Yes)

    ✓ Asked about the onset of pain (Sudden onset)

VINDICATE

Vascular (see PQRST):

    ✓ Asked if I am stationary for long periods of time (No, I am usually active)

    Asked if I have ever had a blood clot (No)

    ✓ Asked if I am short of breath (Not now, but I am with exertion)

Infectious:

    ✓ Asked if I have had a fever or chills (No)

Neoplastic: Not applicable

Degenerative: Not applicable

Immunologic: Not applicable

Congenital: Not applicable

(**A**dded) Toxin/poison/drugs: Not applicable

Trauma: Not applicable

CASE 4 (continued)

Electrolytes/metabolic:

___Asked if the pain is associated with meals (No)

Other history:

Past medical history:

___Asked if I have hypertension, high cholesterol, or diabetes (Hypertension)

Family history:

___Asked about a family history of heart disease (Yes, my father died of a heart attack at age 53)

Social history:

___Asked if I smoke or use alcohol (Quit smoking 10 years ago, no alcohol)

Medication and allergies: Noncontributory

Review of systems: Has nausea, chest pain, shortness of breath, and diaphoresis. No fever, chills, weight loss, headache, fainting, lightheadedness, vomiting, diarrhea, constipation, malaise, or fatigue.

Physical Exam Checklist:

___Washed hands before the exam
___Asked to untie gown

Head and neck:

___Listened to neck with stethoscope (Bilateral carotid bruits)

Chest:

___Observed chest wall for symmetric expansion/contraction (Symmetric expansion and contraction)
___Palpated heart over left ribs (Laterally displaced point of maximal impulse)
___Percussed on back (Resonant throughout)
___Listened to lungs in more than 4 places in the front and back (Lungs clear to auscultation)
___Listened to heart in more than 3 places (Regular rate and rhythm)

Abdomen: Not applicable

Pelvis: Not applicable

Extremities: Not applicable

Skin:

___Observed external chest (No lesions or surgical scars)

Nerves: Not applicable

Psychiatric: Not applicable

You should have gotten at least 19 of the 27 possible checkmarks.

CASE 4 (continued)

YOUR NOTE

Differential Diagnosis (list up to 5 in order of likelihood)

1.

2.

3.

4.

5.

History (including positives and negatives from history of present illness, past medical history, family history, social history, and review of systems)

_____

_____

_____

_____

_____

_____

Physical Exam (consisting of positives and negatives relevant to the chief complaint)

_____

_____

_____

_____

_____

_____

Diagnostic Workup (up to 5 items necessary for further diagnosis)

1.

2.

3.

4.

5.

(see p. 124 for sample note)

CASE 5

Mr. Charles Fisher is a 57-year-old male who has come to see you for knee and hip pain. He is a retired construction worker and the pain is affecting his mobility.

Vital signs:

Temperature: 98.4°F
Blood pressure: 126/82 mmHg
Pulse: 74
Respirations: 14

Upon meeting Mr. Fisher you see that he is an overweight male in no acute distress. You have 15 minutes to take a history and perform a focused physical exam on Mr. Fisher.

PREDICTED CHECKLIST

History Checklist:

_____
_____
_____
_____
_____
_____
_____
_____

Physical Exam Checklist:

_____
_____
_____
_____
_____
_____
_____

CASE 5 (continued)

SAMPLE CHECKLIST

History Checklist:

PQRST

P is for **Provokes**:

✓ Asked if anything makes the pain worse (Physical activity. The pain is worse with walking and standing)

✓ Asked if I had tried treating the pain (Yes, ibuprofen helps the pain somewhat)

Q is for **Quality**:

✓ Asked if pain is sharp, dull, or achy (The pain is dull and it feels like I have gravel in my joints)

R is for **Radiation**:

✓ Asked where the pain is (Both hips and knees, right worse than left)

✓ Asked if the pain radiates (No)

S is for **Severity**:

✓ Asked if the pain limits my physical activity (Yes, it prevents me from walking long distances and climbing stairs like I used to)

✓ Asked me to rate the pain on a scale of 1–10, 10 being the worst (The pain is a 5/10)

T is for **Time**:

✓ Asked how long I have had the pain (It has gotten worse over the last 8 months)

✓ Asked if I have had the pain before (Off and on over the years)

VINDICATE

Vascular (see PQRST): Not applicable

Infectious:

✓ Asked if I have had flu-like symptoms (No)

✓ Asked if I have had Lyme disease (No)

Neoplastic: Not applicable

Degenerative:

✓ Asked me if the joints are stiff in the morning (Yes)

✓ Asked me if the pain is worse with movement (Yes)

Immunologic:

✓ Asked if the joint pain is symmetric (No)

✓ Asked about generalized weakness or fatigue (No)

✓ Asked if joints are warm or swollen (No)

✓ Asked if I have a rash (No)

CASE 5 (continued)

Congenital: Not applicable

(Added) Toxin/poison/drugs: Not applicable

Trauma:

____Asked if I ever injured the joints (Frequent aches and pains with construction work)

Electrolytes/metabolic:

____Asked if I have ever had gout (No)
____Asked if the joints are warm and painful to the touch (No)

Other history:

Past medical history, family history, social history, medication, and allergies: Noncontributory

Review of systems: No fever, chills, headaches, chest pain, shortness of breath nausea, vomiting, diarrhea, constipation, weight loss, malaise, or lethargy.

Physical Exam Checklist:

____Washed hands before the exam
____Asked to untie gown

Head and neck: Not applicable

Abdomen: Not applicable

Pelvis: Not applicable

Extremities:

____Observed external surface of knees, hips, elbows, wrists, and feet (Bilateral quadriceps and gluteal atrophy, no joint redness or swelling)
____Palpated knees, hips, elbows, wrists, and feet (Mild bilateral knee tenderness with firm palpation, no joint warmth, crepitus in knees and hips bilaterally)
____Assessed passive and active range of motion in knees and hips (Limited adduction, abduction, extension, flexion, internal rotation, and external rotation of hips; limited flexion and extension of knees)
____Observed me walking (Antalgic gait favoring left leg)

Skin: Not applicable

Nerves: Not applicable

Psychiatric: Not applicable

You should have gotten at least 18 of the 26 possible checkmarks.

CASE 5 (continued)

YOUR NOTE

Differential Diagnosis (list up to 5 in order of likelihood)

1.

2.

3.

4.

5.

History (including positives and negatives from history of present illness, past medical history, family history, social history, and review of systems)

_____

_____

_____

_____

_____

_____

Physical Exam (consisting of positives and negatives relevant to the chief complaint)

_____

_____

_____

_____

_____

_____

Diagnostic Workup (up to 5 items necessary for further diagnosis)

1.

2.

3.

4.

5.

(see p. 125 for sample note)

CASE 6

Mr. Jacob Miller is a 60-year-old male who has come to see you for a fever and cough.

Vital signs:

Temperature: 102.0°F
Blood pressure: 120/82 mmHg
Pulse: 70
Respirations: 14

Upon meeting Mr. Miller you see that he is ill-appearing and breathing comfortably at rest. You have 15 minutes to take a history and perform a focused physical exam on Mr. Miller.

PREDICTED CHECKLIST

History Checklist:

onset, preceding events (runny nose, headache ...), productive cough? phlegm? aspect? blood? amount? fever? night sweats? SOB? chest pain? abdominal pain? alleviating / exacerbating factors? if pain, severity, radiation, timing? coughing at night? Need additional pillows to sleep? TB contacts? Recent travel? Smoking? drinking, drugs, occupation, sexual activity, PMSH, FH, weight loss, fatigue?

Physical Exam Checklist:

HEENT, neck (JVD, carotid pulse, lymphadenopathy) pulmonary (inspection, palpation, percussion, auscultation), CV (palpation, auscultation) abdominal (inspection, ausc, percussion, ausc) extremities (pulses, lesions, clubbing, cyanosis)

CASE 6 (continued)

SAMPLE CHECKLIST

History Checklist:

PQRST

P is for **Provokes**:

_____Asked if anything makes the cough worse (Nothing really, it's just always there)

_____Asked if I had tried treating the cough (Yes, I have been taking cold medicine that hasn't helped)

Q is for **Quality**:

_____Asked if the cough was dry, productive of sputum, or bloody (Cough started as dry, but now is productive of yellow sputum [Never bloody])

R is for **Radiation**: Not applicable

S is for **Severity**:

_____Asked if I feel short of breath (No)

_____Asked if cough limits my daily activities or keeps me awake (Yes, it keeps me awake, and I have missed the last 2 days at work)

T is for **Time**:

_____Asked how long I had the cough (3 days)

_____Asked about the onset of the cough (Sudden onset after a fever for 1 day)

_____Asked if the cough is constant or intermittent (Cough is constant)

VINDICATE

Vascular:

_____Asked if cough is worse when lying down (No)

Infectious:

_____Asked if I have had a fever or chills (Yes, my temperature has been about 102°F, and I have chills)

_____Asked if I have had night sweats (No)

_____Asked about sick contacts (None)

_____Asked about exposure to tuberculosis (None)

Neoplastic:

_____Asked about weight loss (No)

Degenerative: Not applicable

Immunologic: Not applicable

Congenital: Not applicable

CASE 6 (continued)

(**A**dded) Toxin/poison/drugs:

_____Asked if I smoke (No, never have)
_____Asked about exposure to hazardous material like asbestos or silica (No)

Trauma: Not applicable

Electrolytes/metabolic:

_____Asked if cough is related to meals (No)

Other history:

Past medical history, family history, social history, medications, and allergies: Noncontributory

Review of systems: Has had a sore throat, fatigue and malaise. Denies headaches, chest pain, shortness of breath, nausea, vomiting, diarrhea, or constipation.

Physical Exam Checklist:

_____Washed hands before the exam
_____Asked to untie gown

Head and neck:

_____Palpated for enlarged lymph nodes (None palpable)

Chest:

_____Observed chest wall for symmetric expansion and contraction (Symmetric expansion and contraction)
_____Percussed on my back (Dullness over left lower lobe)
_____Listened to my lungs in more than 4 places in the front and back (Coarse crackles throughout, decreased breath sounds over left lower lobe)
_____Listened to heart in more than 3 places (Regular rate and rhythm)

Abdomen: Not applicable

Pelvis: Not applicable

Extremities: Not applicable

Skin:

_____Checked skin over chest (No skin lesions or scars)

Nerves: Not applicable

Psychiatric: Not applicable

You should have gotten at least 18 of the 25 possible checkmarks.

CASE 6 (continued)

YOUR NOTE

Differential Diagnosis (list up to 5 in order of likelihood)

1. pneumonia
2. bronchitis
3. lung cancer.
4. TB
5.

History (including positives and negatives from history of present illness, past medical history, family history, social history, and review of systems)

60 y.o male presents with fever and cough that started 3 days ago. The cough is productive with yellow sputum. He denies SOB, chest pains, abdominal pain, there are no alleviating or exacerbating factors. He denies exposure to TB. Pt doesn't smoke a drink. PMH, SH, FM all non contributory

Physical Exam (consisting of positives and negatives relevant to the chief complaint)

_____
_____
_____
_____
_____
_____

Diagnostic Workup (up to 5 items necessary for further diagnosis)

1.
2.
3.
4.
5.

(see p. 126 for sample note)

CASE 7

Mrs. Eleanor Jacobson is a 76-year-old female who is brought in urgently by her husband, Mr. John Jacobson, because she is confused and cannot move her right arm and leg.

Vital signs:

Temperature: 98.9°F
Blood pressure: 156/98 mmHg
Pulse: 70
Respirations: 14

Upon meeting the couple you see that the patient is sitting comfortably. She acts surprised to see you and seems completely unaware that anything is wrong. You have 15 minutes to take a history and perform a focused physical exam on Mrs. Jacobson.

PREDICTED CHECKLIST

History Checklist:

_____
_____
_____
_____
_____
_____
_____
_____

Physical Exam Checklist:

_____
_____
_____
_____
_____
_____
_____
_____

CASE 7 (continued)

SAMPLE CHECKLIST

History Checklist:

_____Asked if it was okay if my husband was present before starting the interview (Yes)

PQRST

P is for Provokes:

_____Asked if anything makes the symptoms worse (No)
_____Asked if I had tried treating the symptoms (No)

Q is for Quality: Not applicable

R is for Radiation:

_____Asked if symptoms have changed since their onset (She seemed confused first, then she could not move her leg, and the symptoms appear to be progressing)

S is for Severity: Not applicable

T is for Time:

_____Asked how long the symptoms have been present (3 hours)
_____Asked about the onset of symptoms (Gradual onset)

VINDICATE

Vascular:

_____Asked about a history of atherosclerosis (Yes, she had a heart attack years ago)
_____Asked if I have ever had a blood clot (No)
_____Asked if I have ever lost consciousness (No)

Infectious:

_____Asked if I have had a fever, chills, headache, or a stiff neck. (No)

Neoplastic:

_____Asked if I have blurry vision (No)
_____Asked if I have had seizures (No)
_____Asked about weight loss (No)

Degenerative:

_____Asked if I think my memory is good (Yes)

Immunologic: Not applicable

Congenital: Not applicable

(**A**dded) Toxin/poison/drugs:

_____Asked if I take medication, drugs, or alcohol (I take a cholesterol medication, but no alcohol or drugs)
_____Asked about exposure to chemicals or poison (No)

Trauma:

_____Asked if I have hit my head (No)

CASE 7 (continued)

Electrolytes/metabolic:

_____Asked about diet and fluid intake (No recent changes)

Other history:

Past medical history: The patient smokes cigarettes and has a history of hypertension, hyperlipidemia, atherosclerosis, and one myocardial infarct that occurred years ago. No diabetes.

Family history: No Alzheimer's disease

Social history and allergies: Noncontributory

Review of systems: No headaches, fever, chills, blurry vision, chest pain, shortness of breath, nausea, vomiting, diarrhea, or constipation.

Physical Exam Checklist:

_____Washed hands before the exam
_____Asked to untie gown

Head and neck:

_____Examined head for signs of trauma (No signs of trauma)
_____Listened to neck with stethoscope (Bilateral carotid bruits)

Chest:

_____Listened to my lungs in more than 4 places in the front and back (Lungs clear to auscultation)
_____Listened to heart in more than 3 places (Regular rate and rhythm)

Abdomen: Not applicable

Pelvis: Not applicable

Extremities: Not applicable

Skin: Not applicable

Nerves:

_____Tested cranial nerves 2–12 (Homonymous hemianopia, no right visual gaze. Pupils equally round and reactive to light, symmetric facial sensation and muscle strength, symmetric trapezius and sternocleidomastoid muscle strength, adequate uvula and tongue movement)
_____Tested motor function (Flaccid paralysis of right arm and leg)
_____Tested sensation (Reduced light touch sensation in the right hand and foot. Left hand and foot normal)
_____Tested cerebellum (Adequate alternating finger to nose test)
_____Tested reflexes (Brisk right-sided deep tendon reflexes. Up going right toe. Left reflexes normal)

Psychiatric:

_____Performed screening mental status exam (Alert and oriented to place only. Patient unable to perform the rest of the exam)

You should have gotten at least 21 of the 30 possible checkmarks.

CASE 7 (continued)

YOUR NOTE

Differential Diagnosis (list up to 5 in order of likelihood)

1. thrombosis
2. intracranial hemorrhage.
3. intracranial neoplasm.
4. subdural hematoma.
5. subarachnoid hemorrhage.

History (including positives and negatives from history of present illness, past medical history, family history, social history, and review of systems)

76 y.o F presents with confusion and right sided hemi-
plegia. Sy. started 3 hours ago and have gotten pro-
gressively worse (first confusion, then leg, then arm). She
denies headaches, N/V, seizures, blurred vision,
chestpain, SOB, abdominal pains, neck pain. PMH: MI
a few years ago, HTN, hypercholesterolemia and hyperlipidemia,
atherosclerosis. BM (-) FH: noncontributory. SH: smokes,
NKDA.

Physical Exam (consisting of positives and negatives relevant to the chief complaint)

VS: BP 156/98   HR, RR, Temp WNL
HEENT: eyes: - homonymous hemianopia
               - EOM: difficulty gazing to the right
               - PERRLA
neck: carotid bruits absent, no JVD.
CV: RRR, nl S₁S₂, no murmurs, rubs or gallops.
Pulm: bilaterally CTA.
Neurologic: II, III, IV: as above.
            V: sensory deficit

Diagnostic Workup (up to 5 items necessary for further diagnosis)

1. CBC
2. PT/PTT
3. CT head
4. MRI brain
5. LP.

(see p. 127 for sample note)

CASE 8

Ms. Jennifer Nelson is a 22-year-old female who has made an appointment to see you for urinary frequency, urgency, and pain.

Vital signs:

Temperature: 100.0°F
Blood pressure: 132/88 mmHg
Pulse: 70
Respirations: 16

Upon meeting Ms. Nelson, you see that she is sitting comfortably on the examination table. You have 15 minutes to take a history and perform a focused physical exam on Ms. Nelson.

PREDICTED CHECKLIST

History Checklist:

onset / progression / provoking / alleviating factors / location of the pain / radiation / quality. how frequent? how much? incontinence? fever? CVA pain? chills? abdominal pain? Hematuria? fluid retention; weight change? fatigue? Med? PMH? FH? SH? → tob, EtOH, sexual history, occupation. Allergies.

Physical Exam Checklist:

- Pulmonary auscultation / CV auscultation / extremities / abdominal exam.

PE in PM.

CASE 8 (continued)

SAMPLE CHECKLIST

History Checklist:

PQRST

P is for **Provokes**:

_____Asked if anything makes the pain worse (Urination)
_____Asked if I have tried treating the pain (No)

Q is for **Quality**:

_____Asked if pain is dull, sharp, burning, or achy (Pain is burning)

R is for **Radiation**:

_____Asked where the pain is (Points to suprapubic area)
_____Asked if the pain radiates anywhere or has changed location (No)

S is for **Severity**:

_____Asked me to rate the pain on a scale of 1–10, 10 being the worst
(The pain is 5/10)

T is for **Time**:

_____Asked when the pain started (About 3 days ago)
_____Asked about the onset of symptoms (Gradual onset)

VINDICATE

Vascular: Not applicable

Infectious:

_____Asked if I have had a fever or chills (No)
_____Asked if I have a vaginal discharge, itching, or odor (No)
_____Asked if I have blood in the urine (No)
_____Asked if I have vaginal blisters (No)

Neoplastic: Not applicable

Degenerative: Not applicable

Immunologic:

_____Asked about arthritis and oral or genital ulcers (None)

Congenital: Not applicable

(**A**dded) Toxin/poison/drugs: Not applicable

Trauma: Not applicable

Electrolytes/metabolic:

_____Asked if I have had kidney stones (No)
_____Asked about last menstrual period (2 weeks ago and regular)

CASE 8 (continued)

Other history:

Past medical history

_____Asked if I have ever had a urinary tract infection (Yes, I get them often)

Family history and allergies: Noncontributory

Social history:

_____Asked if I could be pregnant (No, I take a birth control pill)
_____Asked about sexual practices and previous sexually transmitted diseases (I am sexually active with one male partner. No sexually transmitted diseases)

Review of systems: No headache, chest pain, shortness of breath, nausea, vomiting, diarrhea, constipation, vaginal discharge, fatigue, or weight loss.

Physical Exam Checklist:

_____Washed hands before the exam
_____Asked to untie gown

Head and neck: Not applicable

Chest: Not applicable

Abdomen:

_____Observed abdomen for distention (No distention)
_____Palpated lightly and deeply in all quadrants (Mild suprapubic tenderness, normal sized liver and spleen, no masses)
_____Percussed on abdomen (Resonant throughout)
_____Percussed firmly over both kidneys (No tenderness)
_____Listened to abdomen is all quadrants (Normal bowel sounds)

Pelvis: Exam deferred

Extremities: Not applicable

Skin:

_____Checked skin over abdomen (No skin lesions or surgical scars)

Nerves: Not applicable

Psychiatric: Not applicable

You should have gotten at least 19 of the 26 possible checkmarks.

CASE 8 (continued)

YOUR NOTE

Differential Diagnosis (list up to 5 in order of likelihood)

1. lower UTI
2. pyelonephritis.
3. interstitial cystitis
4. lithiasis
5. bladder cancer.

History (including positives and negatives from history of present illness, past medical history, family history, social history, and review of systems)

22 y.o F who presents with urinary frequency, urgency and pain that started 3 days ago. The pain is located in the suprapubic area. She denies any vaginal discharge, itching or odor. She has no fever, chills or hematuria. PMH is significant for recurrent UTI. No history of STD. FH, SH: noncontributory. Meds: OCP, NKDA.

Physical Exam (consisting of positives and negatives relevant to the chief complaint)

HEENT: no oral ulcers.
CV: RRR S₁ S₂, no murmurs, rubs or gallops.
Pulmonary: bilaterally CTA.
Abdomen: soft, nontender, nondistended, BS(+)
Extremities + skin: no lesions or rashes.
— no edema.

Diagnostic Workup (up to 5 items necessary for further diagnosis)

1. genital + pelvic exam.
2. UA + gram stain + culture.
3. CBC
4. renal U/S
5. cervical cultures.

(see p. 128 for sample note)

CASE 9

Mr. James Daniels is a 21-year-old male who made an urgent appointment to see you for a cough, shortness of breath, and chest tightness.

Vital signs:

Temperature: 98.9°F
Blood pressure: 130/86 mmHg
Pulse: 70
Respirations: 24

Upon meeting Mr. Daniels, you see that he is a young man with labored breathing. You have 15 minutes to take a history and perform a focused physical exam on Mr. Daniels.

PREDICTED CHECKLIST

History Checklist:

onset? intermittent/continuous? provoking factors?
relieving factors? sx at night? previous events?
allergies? Meds? Recent exposure? TB contact?
fevers? phlegm? aspect/amount? I chest pain?
Abdominal pain? N/V D/C? sore throat? runny
nose? swollen glands & lymph nodes? recent
weight loss? night sweats? PMH, SH, FH

Physical Exam Checklist:

CASE 9 (continued)

SAMPLE CHECKLIST

History Checklist:

PQRST

P is for Provokes:

____Asked if anything makes the symptoms worse (Exercise. Every time I run I have to stop because I can't breathe. Sometimes, like now, it just happens for no reason)

____Asked if I had tried any treatments (No, but it usually gets better when I rest)

Q is for Quality:

____Asked if the cough was dry, productive of sputum, or bloody (Cough is dry)

R is for Radiation: Not applicable

S is for Severity:

____Asked how long I can exercise without symptoms (Just a few minutes)

T is for Time:

____Asked how long I have had the symptoms (Off and on since childhood, but never this bad)

____Asked if the symptoms are constant or intermittent (The symptoms are intermittent and are completely gone most of the time)

VINDICATE

Vascular:

____Asked if I have ever had a blood clot (No)

____Asked if I have been immobile for a long period of time (No)

Infectious:

____Asked if I have had a fever or chills (No)

Neoplastic:

____Asked about weight loss and fatigue (No)

Degenerative: Not applicable

Immunologic:

____Asked if I have environmental allergies (I have seasonal allergies to pollen in the air)

____Asked if I have wheezes (Yes)

Congenital: Not applicable

CASE 9 (continued)

(**A**dded) Toxin/poison/drugs:

_____Asked if I smoke (No, never have)

_____Asked about exposure to hazardous material like asbestos or silica (No)

_____Asked if I have a carbon monoxide detector in my house (Yes)

Trauma:

_____Asked about trauma to the chest wall (No)

_____Asked about foreign body aspiration (No)

Electrolytes/metabolic: Not applicable

Other history:

Past medical history, family history, social history, and medications: Noncontributory

Review of systems: No headache, sore throat, chest pain, nausea, vomiting, diarrhea, constipation, malaise, or lethargy.

Physical Exam Checklist:

_____Washed hands before the exam

_____Asked to untie gown

Head and neck:

_____Palpated for enlarged lymph nodes (None palpable)

_____Looked in the back of my throat (Normal appearing pharynx and uvula)

Chest:

_____Observed chest wall for symmetric expansion/contraction (Symmetric expansion/contraction)

_____Percussed on my back (Resonant throughout)

_____Listened to lungs in more than 4 places in the front and back (Tachypnea with diffuse expiratory wheezes)

_____Listened to heart in more than 4 places (Regular rate and rhythm)

Abdomen: Not applicable

Pelvis: Not applicable

Extremities: Not applicable

Skin:

_____Checked skin over chest (No skin lesions or scars)

Nerves: Not applicable

Psychiatric: Not applicable

You should have gotten at least 19 of the 26 possible checkmarks.

CASE 9 (continued)

YOUR NOTE

Differential Diagnosis (list up to 5 in order of likelihood)

1. Asthma.
6. CHF
2. URI
3. bronchitis
4. atypical pneumonia
5. panic attack.

History (including positives and negatives from history of present illness, past medical history, family history, social history, and review of systems)

21 y.o M presenting with cough, SOB and chest tightness. He has had similar episodes in the past and symptoms are typically exacerbated with exercise and alleviated with rest. He denies fever, chills, chest pain, abdominal pain, sore throat. The cough is non productive. PMH, FM, Meds, SH non contributory. Allergies: pollen, NKDA.

Physical Exam (consisting of positives and negatives relevant to the chief complaint)

VS: . . .

Pt. in respiratory distress   HEENT: throat: no erythema, or exudate, red ; no cervical lymphadenopathy, no JVD   Pulmonary: bilateral expiratory wheezing, no rales or ronchi   CV: RRR, S₁S₂, no murmurs, rubs or gallops   Extremities: no rashes, no cyanosis, no clubbing

Diagnostic Workup (up to 5 items necessary for further diagnosis)

1. expirator peak flow measurement.
2. ABG
3. CBC
4. EKG
5. PFT

(see p. 129 for sample note)

CASE 10

Ms. Jane Becker is a 21-year-old college student who has come to see you because she is weak and her skin itches.

Vital signs:

Temperature: 100.2°F
Blood pressure: 118/70 mmHg
Pulse: 64
Respirations: 24

Upon meeting Ms. Becker you see that she is jaundiced and scratching her abdomen. You have 15 minutes to take a history and perform a focused physical exam on Ms. Becker.

PREDICTED CHECKLIST

History Checklist:

_____
_____
_____
_____
_____
_____
_____
_____

Physical Exam Checklist:

_____
_____
_____
_____
_____
_____
_____

CASE 10 (continued)

SAMPLE CHECKLIST

History Checklist:

PQRST

P is for **Provokes**:

    _____Asked if anything makes the symptoms worse (No)
    _____Asked if I had tried treating the symptoms (No)

Q is for **Quality**: Not applicable

R is for **Radiation**: Not applicable

S is for **Severity**: Not applicable

T is for **Time**:

    _____Asked how long the symptoms have been present (About 1 week)
    _____Asked about the onset of symptoms (Gradual onset)

VINDICATE

Vascular:

    _____Asked if I am fatigued or light headed (No)
    _____Asked if I have dark colored urine (No)
    _____Asked if I have ever had a blood transfusion (No)

Infectious:

    _____Asked if I have had a fever or chills (Yes, I have had a fever for the last few days)
    _____Asked about abdominal pain (Yes, I have crampy abdominal pain)
    _____Asked about change in bowel movements (I have had diarrhea for about a week)
    _____Asked about nausea and vomiting (Yes, I have felt nauseous)
    _____Asked about camping or recent travel (Yes, I returned from a vacation in Mexico 3 weeks ago)
    _____Asked about sick contacts (None)

Neoplastic:

    _____Asked about weight loss (Yes, I have lost about 8 pounds in the last month. I just haven't had an appetite)

Degenerative: Not applicable

Immunologic:

    _____Asked if I have had hepatitis vaccinations (No)

Congenital:

    _____Asked if I was jaundiced during infancy (I don't think so)

CASE 10 (continued)

(**A**dded) Toxin/poison/drugs:

_____Asked if I take medication, drugs, or alcohol (I take an oral contraceptive and I drink 2 alcoholic drinks per day)
_____Asked about exposure to chemicals or poison (No)

Trauma:

Electrolytes/metabolic: Not applicable

Other history:

Past medical history, family history, medications, and allergies: Noncontributory

Social history:

_____Asked if I am sexually active (Yes with one partner)
_____Asked if I could be pregnant (No, I take an oral contraceptive)

Review of systems: No headache, chest pain, or shortness of breath

Physical Exam Checklist:

_____Washed hands before the exam
_____Asked to untie gown

Head and neck:

_____Examined sclerae (Icteric)
_____Examined pharynx (Normal)
_____Palpated for enlarged lymph nodes (None palpable)

Chest:

_____Listened to my lungs in more than 4 places in the front and back (Lungs clear to auscultation)
_____Listened to heart in more than 3 places (Regular rate and rhythm)

Abdomen:

_____Observed abdomen for distention (No distention)
_____Percussed over liver (Moderately enlarged and tender liver)
_____Palpated lightly and deeply in all quadrants (Mild diffuse abdominal tenderness, normal sized spleen, no masses)
_____Listened to abdomen is all quadrants (Hyperactive bowel sounds)

Pelvis: Not applicable

Extremities: Not applicable

Skin:

_____Examined skin diffusely (Jaundice, no lesions, rashes, or scars)

Nerves: Not applicable

Psychiatric: Not applicable

You should have gotten at least 22 of the 32 possible checkmarks.

CASE 10 (continued)

YOUR NOTE

Differential Diagnosis (list up to 5 in order of likelihood)

1.

2.

3.

4.

5.

History (including positives and negatives from history of present illness, past medical history, family history, social history, and review of systems)

_____

_____

_____

_____

_____

_____

Physical Exam (consisting of positives and negatives relevant to the chief complaint)

_____

_____

_____

_____

_____

_____

Diagnostic Workup (up to 5 items necessary for further diagnosis)

1.

2.

3.

4.

5.

(see p. 130 for sample note)

CASE 11

Mr. John Andrews is a 31-year-old male attorney who has come to see you for headaches. He does not have a headache now, but his last one was 2 days ago. He is otherwise healthy.

Vital signs:

Temperature: 98.7°F
Blood pressure: 124/78 mmHg
Pulse: 64
Respirations: 14

Upon meeting Mr. Andrews you see that he is a healthy-appearing male in no acute distress. You have 15 minutes to take a history and perform a focused physical exam on Mr. Andrews.

PREDICTED CHECKLIST

History Checklist:

_____
_____
_____
_____
_____
_____
_____
_____

Physical Exam Checklist:

_____
_____
_____
_____
_____
_____
_____

CASE 11 (continued)

SAMPLE CHECKLIST

History Checklist:

PQRST

P is for **Provokes**:

_____Asked if anything triggers the headaches (Stress at work seems to make them come on. Bright light, rapid head movements, and coughing makes them worse.)

_____Asked if I had tried treating the symptoms (Ibuprofen, sleep, and darkness seem to help)

Q is for **Quality**:

_____Asked me to describe the headache (The headaches begin as a dull throbbing behind my eyes and progress to a sharp pain and I see flashing lights)

R is for **Radiation**:

_____Asked if the pain is present anywhere else (No)

S is for **Severity**:

_____Asked if the headaches prevent me from working (Yes, I cannot read or see well during the headaches)

_____Asked to rate the pain on a scale of 1–10, 10 being the worst (9/10)

T is for **Time**:

_____Asked when I had my first headache (About 6 months ago)

_____Asked how often the headaches occur (About once every month)

_____Asked how long the headaches last (Usually a few hours, but can last the whole day)

VINDICATE

Vascular:

_____Asked if I have had changes in speech, balance, or memory (No)

Infectious:

_____Asked if I have had a fever, chills, or a stiff neck (No)

_____Asked if I have had a sinus infection (No)

Neoplastic:

_____Asked if I have had seizures (No)

_____Asked if I have lost consciousness (No)

_____Asked about weight loss (No)

Degenerative:

_____Asked if I think my memory is good (Yes)

Immunologic: Not applicable

Congenital: Not applicable

(**A**dded) Toxin/poison/drugs:

_____Asked if I take caffeine, medications, drugs, or alcohol (I have 1 cup of coffee per day. No drugs or alcohol.)

_____Asked if I have a carbon monoxide detector (Yes)

CASE 11 (continued)

Trauma:

_____Asked if I have ever hit my head (No)
_____Asked if I have pain in my temporomandibular joint (No)

Electrolytes/metabolic: Not applicable

Other history:

Past medical history, social history, medications, and allergies: Noncontributory

Family history:

_____Asked if anyone in my family has similar headaches (Yes, my dad)

Review of systems: No sore throat, fever, chills, chest pain, shortness of breath, nausea, vomiting, diarrhea, or constipation.

Physical Exam Checklist:

_____Washed hands before the exam
_____Asked to untie gown

Head and neck:

_____Examined head for signs of trauma (No signs of trauma)
_____Checked for neck stiffness (None)

Chest:

_____Listened to my lungs in more than 4 places in the front and back (Lungs clear to auscultation)
_____Listened to heart in more than 3 places (Regular rate and rhythm)

Abdomen: Not applicable

Pelvis: Not applicable

Extremities: Not applicable

Skin: Not applicable

Nerves:

_____Tested cranial nerves 2–12 (Vision adequate, pupils equally round and reactive to light, extraocular muscles intact, symmetric facial sensation and muscle strength, symmetric trapezius and sternocleidomastoid muscle strength, adequate uvula and tongue movement)
_____Tested motor function (Adequate and symmetric strength in all extremities)
_____Tested sensation (Adequate and symmetric light touch sensation in all extremities)
_____Tested cerebellum (No gait abnormalities, adequate alternating finger to nose test)
_____Tested reflexes (Reflexes adequate and symmetric)

Psychiatric:

_____Performed screening mental status exam (No deficiencies in attention, orientation, memory, abstract thinking, following commands, language usage, or problem solving)
_____Asked about my mood and feelings of depression (Mood okay, not depressed)

You should have gotten at least 24 of the 34 possible checkmarks.

CASE 11 (continued)

YOUR NOTE

Differential Diagnosis (list up to 5 in order of likelihood)

1.

2.

3.

4.

5.

History (including positives and negatives from history of present illness, past medical history, family history, social history, and review of systems)

_____

_____

_____

_____

_____

_____

Physical Exam (consisting of positives and negatives relevant to the chief complaint)

_____

_____

_____

_____

_____

_____

Diagnostic Workup (up to 5 items necessary for further diagnosis)

1.

2.

3.

4.

5.

(see p. 131 for sample note)

CASE 12

Mrs. Joan Jackson is a 54-year-old G4 P4 female who has come to see you for postcoital spotting. She lives 4 hours from town and doesn't see a doctor regularly. Her husband of 30 years, Mr. Ronald Jackson, is with her.

Vital signs:

Temperature: 98.5°F
Blood pressure: 126/84 mmHg
Pulse: 68
Respirations: 16

Upon meeting the couple, you see that the patient is moderately over-weight and sitting comfortably on the examination table. You have 15 minutes to take a history and perform a focused physical exam on Mrs. Jackson.

PREDICTED CHECKLIST

History Checklist:

_____

_____

_____

_____

_____

_____

_____

_____

Physical Exam Checklist:

_____

_____

_____

_____

_____

_____

_____

_____

CASE 12 (continued)

SAMPLE CHECKLIST

History Checklist:

_____Asked if it was okay for my husband to be present before starting the interview (Yes)

PQRST

P is for Provokes:

_____Asked if anything makes the bleeding worse (It only happens after sex)

_____Asked if I had tried any treatments (No)

Q is for Quality: Not applicable

R is for Radiation: Not applicable

S is for Severity:

_____Asked me how much I bleed (Not a lot, just a few spots of blood)

_____Asked if I ever feel light-headed or fatigued (No)

T is for Time:

_____Asked when the bleeding started (About 5 months ago)

_____Asked if it happens every time I have sex (Not at first, but now it does)

VINDICATE

Vascular:

_____Asked about a history of bleeding problems (No)

Infectious:

_____Asked if I have pain with intercourse (No)

_____Asked if I have had a fever or chills (No)

_____Asked about vaginal discharge (Yes, the blood and yellow mucous)

_____Asked about vaginal odor (Yes, sometimes the discharge smells bad)

_____Asked about pain or bleeding with urination (No)

Neoplastic:

_____Asked when I had my last Pap smear (I can't remember, it's been years)

_____Asked if I ever had an abnormal Pap smear (Yes, but I can't remember the results)

_____Asked about blood in the stool (No)

Degenerative:

_____Asked if I have vaginal itching (No)

Immunologic: Not applicable

Congenital: Not applicable

(Added) Toxin/poison/drugs:

_____Asked if I smoke (Yes, about half a pack per day for the last 20 years)

CASE 12 (continued)

Trauma: Not applicable

Electrolytes/metabolic:

_____Asked about last menstrual period (Menopause at age 50, last period 4 years ago)

Other history:

Past medical history, family history, and allergies: Noncontributory

Social:

_____Asked about sexual partners (Just my husband)

_____Asked about sexual practices (Penile-vaginal sex only, nothing unusually rough)

_____Asked about previous sexually transmitted diseases (None)

Medications:

_____Asked if I am taking hormone replacement therapy (No)

Review of systems:

Denies headache, chest pain, shortness of breath, nausea, vomiting, diarrhea, constipation, fatigue, or weight loss

Physical Exam Checklist:

_____Washed hands before the exam

_____Asked to untie gown

Head and neck: Not applicable

Chest:

_____Listened to lungs in more than 4 places in front and back (Lungs clear to auscultation)

_____Listened to heart in more than 3 places (Regular rate and rhythm)

Abdomen:

_____Observed abdomen for distention (None)

_____Palpated lightly and deeply in all quadrants (Nontender, normal sized liver and spleen, no masses)

_____Percussed on abdomen (Resonant throughout)

_____Percussed firmly over both kidneys (No tenderness)

_____Listened to abdomen in all quadrants (Active bowel sounds)

Pelvis: Exam deferred

Extremities:

_____Palpated inguinal lymph nodes (Numerous matted, immobile nodes present)

Skin:

_____Checked skin for bruising/signs of bleeding (No bruises or lesions)

Nerves: Not applicable

Psychiatric: Not applicable

You should have gotten at least 24 of the 34 possible checkmarks.

CASE 12 (continued)

YOUR NOTE

Differential Diagnosis (list up to 5 in order of likelihood)

1.

2.

3.

4.

5.

History (including positives and negatives from history of present illness, past medical history, family history, social history, and review of systems)

_____

_____

_____

_____

_____

_____

Physical Exam (consisting of positives and negatives relevant to the chief complaint)

_____

_____

_____

_____

_____

_____

Diagnostic Workup (up to 5 items necessary for further diagnosis)

1.

2.

3.

4.

5.

(see p. 132 for sample note)

CASE 13

Mrs. Mary Evans is a 24-year-old G2 P1 female at 31 weeks gestation who has come to see you for vaginal bleeding.

Vital signs:

Temperature: 98.8°F
Blood pressure: 128/86 mmHg
Pulse: 74
Respirations: 16
Fetal heart rate: 140

Upon meeting Mrs. Evans, you see a pregnant female sitting comfortably on the examination table. You have 15 minutes to take a history and perform a focused physical exam on Mrs. Evans.

PREDICTED CHECKLIST

History Checklist:

_____
_____
_____
_____
_____
_____
_____
_____

Physical Exam Checklist:

_____
_____
_____
_____
_____
_____
_____
_____

CASE 13 (continued)

SAMPLE CHECKLIST

History Checklist:

PQRST

P is for **Provokes**:

_____Asked if anything makes the bleeding worse (I first noticed it after having sex about 2 weeks ago)

_____Asked if I had tried any treatments (No)

Q is for **Quality**:

_____Asked if the blood is bright red (Yes, with some dark red semisolid material in it)

_____Asked if I had any pain with the bleeding (No)

R is for **Radiation**: Not applicable

S is for **Severity**:

_____Asked me how much I bleed (Started as a few spots occasionally, but now there is much more blood)

_____Asked if I ever feel light-headed or fatigued (I have felt fatigued since I became pregnant)

T is for **Time**:

_____Asked when the bleeding started (About 2 weeks ago after sexual intercourse)

_____Asked how often bleeding occurs (Almost daily)

VINDICATE

Vascular:

_____Asked about a history of bleeding problems during and before pregnancy (No)

Infectious:

_____Asked if I have had a fever or chills (No)

_____Asked about vaginal discharge (Just the blood and clots)

_____Asked about pain or bleeding with urination (No)

Neoplastic:

_____Asked about last Pap smear (About a year ago and it was normal)

Degenerative: Not applicable

Immunologic: Not applicable

Congenital: Not applicable

(**A**dded) Toxin/poison/drugs:

_____Asked if I smoke or use drugs and alcohol (No)

Trauma:

_____Asked about trauma to the abdomen or pelvis (No)

CASE 13 (continued)

Electrolytes/metabolic:

_____Asked if I have had uterine contractions (No)
_____Asked if I have had leakage of amniotic fluid (No)

Other history:

Past medical history, family history, and allergies: Noncontributory

Medications: Prenatal vitamins

Social:

_____Asked about previous sexually transmitted diseases (None)

Review of systems:

Denies headache, chest pain, shortness of breath, nausea, vomiting, diarrhea, or constipation

Physical Exam Checklist:

_____Washed hands before the exam
_____Asked to untie gown

Head and neck: Not applicable

Chest:

_____Listened to lungs in more than 4 places in the front and back (Lungs clear to auscultation)
_____Listened to heart in more than 3 places (Regular rate and rhythm)

Abdomen:

_____Observed abdomen for distention (Consistent with pregnancy)
_____Palpated lightly (no deep palpation) in all quadrants (Fundal height consistent with gestational age, normal sized liver and spleen, no masses)
_____Palpated uterus for fetal position (Longitudinal lie, cephalic presentation)
_____Assessed fetal heart sounds with a Doppler monitor (Audible fetal hearts tones, normal rate)
_____Listened to abdomen in all quadrants (Active bowel sounds)

Pelvis: Exam deferred

Extremities: Not applicable

Skin:

_____Checked skin everywhere for bruising/signs of bleeding (No lesions, bruises, or rashes)

Nerves: Not applicable

Psychiatric: Not applicable

You should have gotten at least 20 of the 28 possible checkmarks.

CASE 13 (continued)

YOUR NOTE

Differential Diagnosis (list up to 5 in order of likelihood)

1.

2.

3.

4.

5.

History (including positives and negatives from history of present illness, past medical history, family history, social history, and review of systems)

_____

_____

_____

_____

_____

_____

Physical Exam (consisting of positives and negatives relevant to the chief complaint)

_____

_____

_____

_____

_____

_____

Diagnostic Workup (up to 5 items necessary for further diagnosis)

1.

2.

3.

4.

5.

(see p. 133 for sample note)

CASE 14

Mr. James Jensen is a 60-year-old male who has made an urgent appointment to see you for foot pain.

Vital signs:

Temperature: 101.0°F
Blood pressure: 126/82 mmHg
Pulse: 72
Respirations: 14

Upon meeting Mr. Jensen you see that he is obese, diaphoretic, and sitting on the examination table with his left shoe off. You have 15 minutes to take a history and perform a focused physical exam on Mr. Jensen.

PREDICTED CHECKLIST

History Checklist:

_____

_____

_____

_____

_____

_____

_____

_____

Physical Exam Checklist:

_____

_____

_____

_____

_____

_____

_____

_____

CASE 14 (continued)

SAMPLE CHECKLIST

History Checklist:

PQRST

P is for **Provokes**:

_____Asked if anything makes the pain worse (Everything. The pain is there all the time and the slightest movement sets it off.)

_____Asked if I had tried treating the pain (Yes, ibuprofen does not help)

Q is for **Quality**:

_____Asked if pain is sharp, dull, crushing, or achy (The pain is crushing)

R is for **Radiation**:

_____Asked where the pain is located (It started in my big toe and now involves the whole foot)

S is for **Severity**:

_____Asked if the pain limited physical activity (Yes, it prevents me from walking, working, and I can't sleep)

_____Asked me to rate the pain on a scale of 1–10, 10 being the worst (The pain is 10/10)

T is for **Time**:

_____Asked how long I have had the pain (About 1 day)

_____Asked if I have had similar pain before (No)

_____Asked about the onset of pain (Gradual onset)

VINDICATE

Vascular (see **PQRST**):

_____Asked about prior blood clots or peripheral vascular disease (No)

Infectious:

_____Asked if I have had a fever or chills (Yes, my temperature has been about 102°F)

_____Asked if I have had flu-like symptoms and a rash (No)

_____Asked if I have ever had Lyme disease (No)

_____Asked if the toe is warm and painful to the touch (Yes)

Neoplastic: Not applicable

Degenerative:

_____Asked if I have pain in other joints (No)

Immunologic: Not applicable

Congenital: Not applicable

(**A**dded) Toxin/poison/drugs: Not applicable

CASE 14 (continued)

Trauma:

      ____Asked if I injured the toe/foot (No)

Electrolytes/metabolic:

      ____Asked if I have ever had gout (No)

Other history:

Past medical history, family history, allergies, social history and medication: Noncontributory

Review of systems: Denies headaches, chest pain, shortness of breath, nausea, vomiting, diarrhea, constipation, or weight loss.

Physical Exam Checklist:

      ____Washed hands before the exam

      ____Asked to untie gown

Head and neck: Not applicable

Chest:

      ____Listened to lungs in more than 4 places front and back (Lungs clear to auscultation)

      ____Listened to heart in more than 3 places (Regular rate and rhythm)

Abdomen: Not applicable

Pelvis: Not applicable

Extremities:

      ____Examined external surface of both feet, knees, and hips (Left toe and foot red and swollen with tense, shiny skin. All other joints are normal.)

      ____Palpated right foot, both knees and hips, and assessed range of motion (Nontender joints, adequate range of motion)

      ____Palpated left foot and great toe lightly (Extreme tenderness in toe and foot)

Skin:

      ____Observed skin over trunk and abdomen (No rash)

Nerves: Not applicable

Psychiatric:

      ____Asked if I am coping with the pain okay (It really hurts bad)

You should have gotten at least 18 of the 26 possible checkmarks.

CASE 14 (continued)

YOUR NOTE

Differential Diagnosis (list up to 5 in order of likelihood)

1.

2.

3.

4.

5.

History (including positives and negatives from history of present illness, past medical history, family history, social history, and review of systems)

_____

_____

_____

_____

_____

_____

Physical Exam (consisting of positives and negatives relevant to the chief complaint)

_____

_____

_____

_____

_____

_____

Diagnostic Workup (up to 5 items necessary for further diagnosis)

1.

2.

3.

4.

5.

(see p. 134 for sample note)

CASE 15

Mr. Peter Watson is a 72-year-old male who has come to see you because he is having trouble urinating.

Vital signs:

Temperature: 98.7°F
Blood pressure: 132/74 mmHg
Pulse: 70
Respirations: 14

Upon meeting Mr. Watson you see that he is moderately overweight and sitting comfortably on the examination table. You have 15 minutes to take a history and perform a focused physical exam on Mr. Watson.

PREDICTED CHECKLIST

History Checklist:

_____
_____
_____
_____
_____
_____
_____
_____

Physical Exam Checklist:

_____
_____
_____
_____
_____
_____
_____

CASE 15 (continued)

SAMPLE CHECKLIST

History Checklist:

PQRST

P is for Provokes:

_____Asked if anything makes the symptoms worse (Drinking a lot of water)

_____Asked if I had tried any treatments (No, but if I strain I can empty my bladder)

Q is for Quality:

_____Asked if I feel like my bladder is still full after I urinate (Yes)

_____Asked if I have a good stream of urine (No, it just drips out)

_____Asked if I ever have to rush to the bathroom to urinate (Yes)

R is for Radiation: Not applicable

S is for Severity: Not applicable

T is for Time:

_____Asked when the symptoms began (About 6 weeks ago)

_____Asked me how often I need to urinate (More than I used to. It seems like I always have to go and when I do very little comes out.)

_____Asked if I have to get up at night to urinate (Yes, usually a couple of times)

VINDICATE

Vascular: Not applicable

Infectious:

_____Asked if I have had a fever or chills (No)

_____Asked if it hurts or burns when I urinate (No)

_____Asked about pain or bleeding with urination (No)

Neoplastic:

_____Asked if I have ever had a prostate exam (Yes, years ago, but I can't remember the results)

Degenerative: Not applicable

Immunologic: Not applicable

Congenital: Not applicable

(Added) Toxin/poison/drugs:

_____Asked if I take a diuretic (No)

_____Asked if I drink coffee or alcohol (1 cup of coffer per day. No alcohol)

_____Asked if I take herbal supplements (No)

Trauma: Not applicable

CASE 15 (continued)

Electrolytes/metabolic:

_____Asked about loss of bladder or bowel control (No)

_____Asked if I have diabetes (No)

Other history:

Past medical history, family history, medications, and allergies:
Noncontributory

Social:

_____Asked if I am sexually active (No)

_____Asked about previous sexually transmitted diseases (None)

Review of systems: Denies fever, chills, headache, chest pain, shortness of
breath, nausea, vomiting, diarrhea, constipation, fatigue, or weight loss.

Physical Exam Checklist:

_____Washed hands before the exam

_____Asked to untie gown

Head and neck: Not applicable

Chest: Not applicable

Abdomen:

_____Observed abdomen for distention (None)

_____Palpated lightly and deeply in all quadrants (Nontender, bladder
dome palpable, normal sized liver and spleen, no masses)

_____Percussed on abdomen (Resonant throughout)

_____Percussed firmly over both kidneys (No tenderness)

_____Listened to abdomen in all quadrants (Active bowel sounds)

Pelvis: Not applicable

Extremities: Not applicable

Skin:

_____Observed skin over trunk and abdomen (No lesions)

Nerves:

_____Tested motor function in lower extremities (Strength symmetric and
adequate)

_____Tested sensation in lower extremities (Light touch sensation intact)

Psychiatric: Not applicable

You should have gotten at least 20 of the 29 possible checkmarks.

CASE 15 (continued)

YOUR NOTE

Differential Diagnosis (list up to 5 in order of likelihood)

1.

2.

3.

4.

5.

History (including positives and negatives from history of present illness, past medical history, family history, social history, and review of systems)

_____

_____

_____

_____

_____

_____

Physical Exam (consisting of positives and negatives relevant to the chief complaint)

_____

_____

_____

_____

_____

_____

Diagnostic Workup (up to 5 items necessary for further diagnosis)

1.

2.

3.

4.

5.

(see p. 135 for sample note)

CASE 16

Mr. John Huggins is a 36-year-old male truck driver who has come to see you for pain and swelling in his left lower leg. He just returned from a cross-country drive in his truck. He is otherwise healthy.

Vital signs:

Temperature: 98.6°F
Blood pressure: 138/74 mmHg
Pulse: 68
Respirations: 14

Upon meeting Mr. Huggins you see that he is sitting comfortably. You have 15 minutes to take a history and perform a focused physical exam on Mr. Huggins.

PREDICTED CHECKLIST

History Checklist:

_____
_____
_____
_____
_____
_____
_____
_____

Physical Exam Checklist:

_____
_____
_____
_____
_____
_____
_____
_____

CASE 16 (continued)

SAMPLE CHECKLIST

History Checklist:

PQRST

P is for **Provokes**:

_____Asked if anything makes the pain worse (Walking or flexing my calf muscle)

_____Asked if I had tried treating the symptoms (No)

Q is for **Quality**:

_____Asked me to describe the pain (I feel pressure like my leg muscles are tight)

R is for **Radiation**:

_____Asked if the pain is present anywhere else (No)

S is for **Severity**:

_____Asked to rate the pain on a scale of 1–10, 10 being the worst (4/10)

T is for **Time**:

_____Asked when I first noticed the pain and swelling (Yesterday, right after getting out of my truck)

_____Asked if the pain and swelling are constant or intermittent (Constant, and the swelling seems to be getting worse)

VINDICATE

Vascular:

_____Asked if I have chest pain (No)

_____Asked if I have shortness of breath (No)

_____Asked if I have had a blood clot before (No)

Infectious:

_____Asked if I have had a fever or chills (No)

Neoplastic:

_____Asked if have ever had a tumor (No)

Degenerative: Not applicable

Immunologic: Not applicable

Congenital: Not applicable

(Added) Toxin/poison/drugs:

_____Asked if I smoke (Yes, 1 pack per day)

Trauma:

_____Asked if I injured my leg (No)

CASE 16 (continued)

Electrolytes/metabolic:

_____Asked how long I drive without stopping to walk (Usually about 5 hours at a time)

Other history:

Past medical history, social history, medications, and allergies: Noncontributory

Family history:

_____Asked if anyone in my family has had a blood clot (I don't know)

Review of systems: No headache, fever, chills, chest pain, shortness of breath, nausea, vomiting, diarrhea, or constipation.

Physical Exam Checklist:

_____Washed hands before the exam
_____Asked to untie gown

Head and neck: Not applicable

Chest:

_____Listened to my lungs in more than 4 places in the front and back (Lungs clear to auscultation)
_____Listened to heart in more than 4 places (Regular rate and rhythm)

Abdomen: Not applicable

Pelvis: Not applicable

Extremities:

_____Observed left lower leg and compared it to the right (Left leg is erythematous and swollen from toe to knee with moderate pitting edema. Right leg is normal)
_____Palpated both lower legs (Left leg is tender and warm. Right leg is normal)
_____Checked pulses in both lower legs (Dorsalis pedis pulses are palpable bilaterally)
_____Dorsiflexed both feet (Pain is elicited in the left calf)

Skin: Not applicable

Nerves: Not applicable

Psychiatric: Not applicable

You should have gotten at least 17 of the 24 possible checkmarks.

CASE 16 (continued)

YOUR NOTE

Differential Diagnosis (list up to 5 in order of likelihood)

1.

2.

3.

4.

5.

History (including positives and negatives from history of present illness, past medical history, family history, social history, and review of systems)

_____

_____

_____

_____

_____

_____

Physical Exam (consisting of positives and negatives relevant to the chief complaint)

_____

_____

_____

_____

_____

_____

Diagnostic Workup (up to 5 items necessary for further diagnosis)

1.

2.

3.

4.

5.

(see p. 136 for sample note)

CASE 17

Mr. Joseph Thomas is a 52-year-old male who has come to see you for burning chest pain.

Vital signs:

Temperature: 99.0°F
Blood pressure: 146/38 mmHg
Pulse: 78
Respirations: 16

Upon meeting Mr. Thomas you see that he is sitting comfortably on the examination table. You have 15 minutes to take a history and perform a focused physical exam on Mr. Thomas.

PREDICTED CHECKLIST

History Checklist:

_____
_____
_____
_____
_____
_____
_____
_____

Physical Exam Checklist:

_____
_____
_____
_____
_____
_____
_____

CASE 17 (continued)

SAMPLE CHECKLIST

History Checklist:

PQRST

P is for **Provokes**:

_____Asked what makes the pain worse (Whiskey and coffee)

_____Asked me if anything makes the pain better (It seems to improve after a light bland meal, antacids help too)

Q is for **Quality**:

_____Asked me if pain is sharp, dull, crushing, or achy (The pain is a burning dull ache)

R is for **Radiation**:

_____Asked where the pain is located (He points to a spot in his midepigastric region)

_____Asked if the pain radiates anywhere (No)

S is for **Severity**:

_____Asked me to rate the pain on a scale of 1–10, 10 being the worst (The pain is 6/10)

T is for **Time**:

_____Asked how long I have had the pain (About 1 month)

_____Asked if the pain is constant or intermittent (Intermittent, it seems to come on worse at night sometimes)

VINDICATE

Vascular (see **PQRST**):

_____Asked if I have dark stools (Yes, once in a while)

_____Asked if I feel light-headed or fatigued (No)

_____Asked if I have ever vomited blood (No)

Infectious:

_____Asked if I have had a fever or chills (No)

_____Asked if I have had nausea, vomiting, or diarrhea (No)

Neoplastic:

_____Asked if I have had weight loss or night sweats (No)

Degenerative: Not applicable

Immunologic: Not applicable

Congenital: Not applicable

CASE 17 (continued)

(**A**dded) Toxin/poison/drugs:

_____Asked if I smoke (Yes, about a half pack per day)

_____Asked if I use alcohol (Yes, I have about 3 drinks per night)

_____Asked if I take aspirin or NSAIDs (Yes, I have arthritis and NSAIDs help with the pain)

Trauma: Not applicable

Electrolytes/metabolic: Not applicable

Other history:

Past medical history, family history, social history, medications, allergies: Noncontributory

Review of systems: No headache, fever or chills, shortness of breath, nausea, vomiting, diarrhea, or constipation.

Physical Exam Checklist:

_____Washed hands before the exam

_____Asked to untie gown

Head and neck: Not applicable

Chest:

_____Listened to lungs more than 4 places in the front and back (Lungs clear to auscultation)

_____Listened to heart in more than 3 places (Regular rate and rhythm)

Abdomen:

_____Observed abdomen for distention (None)

_____Palpated lightly and deeply in all quadrants (Mild midepigastic tenderness with deep palpation, normal sized liver and spleen, no masses)

_____Listened to abdomen (Normal bowel sounds)

Pelvis: Not applicable

Extremities: Not applicable

Skin:

_____Observed skin over abdomen (No lesions)

Nerves: Not applicable

Psychiatric: Not applicable

You should have gotten at least 18 of the 25 possible checkmarks.

CASE 17 (continued)

YOUR NOTE

Differential Diagnosis (list up to 5 in order of likelihood)

1.

2.

3.

4.

5.

History (including positives and negatives from history of present illness, past medical history, family history, social history, and review of systems)

_____

_____

_____

_____

_____

_____

Physical Exam (consisting of positives and negatives relevant to the chief complaint)

_____

_____

_____

_____

_____

_____

Diagnostic Workup (up to 5 items necessary for further diagnosis)

1.

2.

3.

4.

5.

(see p. 137 for sample note)

CASE 18

Mr. Joshua Thompson is a 45-year-old male who has come to see you for lower back pain. He is otherwise healthy.

Vital signs:

Temperature: 98.6°F
Blood pressure: 130/80 mmHg
Pulse: 74
Respirations: 14

Upon meeting Mr. Thompson you see that he is sitting comfortably. You have 15 minutes to take a history and perform a focused physical exam on Mr. Thompson.

PREDICTED CHECKLIST

History Checklist:

_____
_____
_____
_____
_____
_____
_____
_____

Physical Exam Checklist:

_____
_____
_____
_____
_____
_____
_____
_____

CASE 18 (continued)

SAMPLE CHECKLIST

History Checklist:

PQRST

P is for **Provokes**:

_____Asked if anything makes the pain worse (Lifting heavy things, sudden unpredicted movements, and sitting for a long time)

_____Asked if I had tried treating the symptoms (I rest and take aspirin, which helps a little)

Q is for **Quality**:

_____Asked me if the pain is sharp, dull, throbbing, or achy (The pain is a dull ache)

R is for **Radiation**:

_____Asked where the pain is located (Points to the center of his back in the lower lumbar area)

_____Asked if the pain is present anywhere else (Yes, there is sometimes pain and numbness down into my left foot)

S is for **Severity**:

_____Asked to rate the pain on a scale of 1–10, 10 being the worst (5/10)

_____Asked if I have ever lost control of bowel or bladder function (No)

T is for **Time**:

_____Asked when I first noticed the pain (I have had some pain for about a year, but it got very bad yesterday after moving some heavy boxes)

_____Asked if the pain and swelling are constant or intermittent (Constant with occasional flare-ups like the one I am having now)

VINDICATE

Vascular: Not applicable

Infectious:

_____Asked if I have had a fever or chills (No)

Neoplastic:

_____Asked if have ever had a tumor (No)

Degenerative:

_____Asked if I have arthritis (No)

Immunologic:

_____Asked if I have pain in other joints (No)

Congenital: Not applicable

(**A**dded) Toxin/poison/drugs: Not applicable

CASE 18 (continued)

Trauma:

_____Asked if I injured my back (Just wear and tear, no specific injury)

Electrolytes/metabolic: not applicable

Other history:

Past medical history, family history, social history, medications, and allergies: Noncontributory

Review of systems: No headache, fever, chills, chest pain, shortness of breath, nausea, vomiting, diarrhea, or constipation.

Physical Exam Checklist:

_____Washed hands before the exam
_____Asked to untie gown

Head and neck: Not applicable

Chest:

_____Listened to lungs in more than 4 places in the front and back (Lungs clear to auscultation)
_____Listened to heart in more than 3 places (Regular rate and rhythm)

Abdomen: Not applicable

Pelvis: Not applicable

Extremities:

_____Observed left lower leg and compared it to the right (Symmetric, no muscle atrophy)
_____Assessed range of motion in spine (Pain with bending backwards)

Skin: Not applicable

Nerves:

_____Assessed sensation in both lower legs (Reduced light touch sensation in left foot)
_____Assessed strength in lower extremities (Reduced plantar flexion strength in left foot)
_____Asked me to walk (No gait abnormalities)
_____Checked all reflexes in lower extremities (Normal, symmetric reflexes)

Psychiatric: Not applicable

You should have gotten at least 17 of the 24 possible checkmarks.

CASE 18 (continued)

YOUR NOTE

Differential Diagnosis (list up to 5 in order of likelihood)

1.

2.

3.

4.

5.

History (including positives and negatives from history of present illness, past medical history, family history, social history, and review of systems)

_____

_____

_____

_____

_____

_____

Physical Exam (consisting of positives and negatives relevant to the chief complaint)

_____

_____

_____

_____

_____

_____

Diagnostic Workup (up to 5 items necessary for further diagnosis)

1.

2.

3.

4.

5.

(see p. 138 for sample note)

CASE 19

Ms. Maria Baker is a 20-year-old G2 Ab1 female who has come to see you for abdominal pain and vaginal bleeding. She is at 8 weeks gestation by last menstrual period.

Vital signs:

Temperature: 98.0°F
Blood pressure: 116/80 mmHg
Pulse: 68
Respirations: 14
Fetal heart tones: Not detectable

Upon meeting Ms. Baker you see a healthy-appearing patient sitting on the examination table holding her lower abdomen. Mr. Joseph Roberts, the patient's boyfriend and the father of the baby, is present. You have 15 minutes to take a history and perform a focused physical exam on Ms. Baker.

PREDICTED CHECKLIST

History Checklist:

_____
_____
_____
_____
_____
_____
_____

Physical Exam Checklist:

_____
_____
_____
_____
_____
_____
_____

CASE 19 (continued)

SAMPLE CHECKLIST

History Checklist:

_____Asked if it was okay for my boyfriend to be present before starting the interview (Yes)

PQRST

P is for **Provokes**:

_____Asked if anything makes the pain better or worse (No, it is constant and unchanged since its onset)

_____Asked if I tried treating the pain (No)

Q is for **Quality**:

_____Asked where the pain is located (Points to left side of lower abdomen/pelvis)

_____Asked if the blood is bright red or dark, clotted blood (Bright red)

_____Asked if the pain is sharp, dull, crampy, or burning (The pain is sharp)

R is for **Radiation**:

_____Asked if the pain radiates anywhere (My upper back/shoulders)

S is for **Severity**:

_____Asked me to rate the pain on a scale of 1–10, 10 being the worst (6/10)

_____Asked me how much I have bled (Not a lot, just a few spots of blood)

_____Asked if I feel light-headed or fatigued (No)

T is for **Time**:

_____Asked when the bleeding started (About 2 hours ago)

_____Asked about the onset of pain and bleeding (Sudden onset)

VINDICATE

Vascular:

_____Asked about a history of bleeding problems (No)

Infectious:

_____Asked if I have had a fever or chills (No)

_____Asked about vaginal discharge (No)

_____Asked about unusual vaginal odor (No)

_____Asked about pain or bleeding with urination (No)

Neoplastic:

_____Asked when I had my last Pap smear (6 months ago, it was normal)

Degenerative: Not applicable

Immunologic: Not applicable

Congenital: Not applicable

(Added) Toxin/poison/drugs: Not applicable

CASE 19 (continued)

Trauma:

    ____Asked about recent trauma (No)
    ____Asked about pain with sexual intercourse (No)

Electrolytes/metabolic:

    ____Asked about last menstrual period (8 weeks ago and regular)

Other history:

Past medical history, family history, medication, and allergies: Noncontributory

Social:

    ____Asked about sexual partners (Just my boyfriend)
    ____Asked about contraception (None)
    ____Asked about sexual practices (Penile-vaginal sex, nothing unusually rough)
    ____Asked about recent intercourse (last time was 1 week ago)
    ____Asked about previous sexually transmitted diseases (I had gonorrhea once several years ago)

Review of systems: Denies headache, fatigue, chest pain, shortness of breath, nausea, vomiting, diarrhea, or constipation.

Physical Exam Checklist:

    ____Washed hands before the exam
    ____Asked to untie gown

Head and neck: Not applicable

Chest:

    ____Listened to lungs in more than 4 places in the front and back (Lungs clear to auscultation)
    ____Listened to heart in more than 3 places (Regular rate and rhythm)

Abdomen:

    ____Observed abdomen for distention (None)
    ____Palpated lightly and deeply in all quadrants (Moderately tender in left lower quadrant with deep palpation, normal sized liver and spleen, uterus nonpalpable, no masses)
    ____Percussed on abdomen (Resonant throughout)
    ____Percussed firmly over both kidneys (No tenderness)
    ____Listened to abdomen is all quadrants (Active bowel sounds)

Pelvis: Exam deferred

Extremities: Not applicable

Skin:

    ____Checked skin everywhere for bruising/signs of bleeding (No skin lesions or bruises)

Nerves: Not applicable

Psychiatric: Not applicable

You should have gotten at least 26 of the 36 possible checkmarks.

CASE 19 (continued)

YOUR NOTE

Differential Diagnosis (list up to 5 in order of likelihood)

1.

2.

3.

4.

5.

History (including positives and negatives from history of present illness, past medical history, family history, social history, and review of systems)

_____

_____

_____

_____

_____

_____

Physical Exam (consisting of positives and negatives relevant to the chief complaint)

_____

_____

_____

_____

_____

_____

Diagnostic Workup (up to 5 items necessary for further diagnosis)

1.

2.

3.

4.

5.

(see p. 139 for sample note)

CASE 20

Mrs. Jennifer Peterson is a 46-year-old female who has come to see you for nausea, vomiting, and abdominal pain.

Vital signs:

Temperature: 98.7°F
Blood pressure: 132/72 mmHg
Pulse: 72
Respirations: 14

Upon meeting Mrs. Peterson you see that she is an obese, diaphoretic female with obvious discomfort. You have 15 minutes to take a history and perform a focused physical exam on Mrs. Peterson.

PREDICTED CHECKLIST

History Checklist:

_____

_____

_____

_____

_____

_____

_____

_____

Physical Exam Checklist:

_____

_____

_____

_____

_____

_____

_____

CASE 20 (continued)

SAMPLE CHECKLIST

History Checklist:

PQRST

P is for **Provokes**:

_____Asked if anything makes the pain worse (It seems worse after I eat)
_____Asked me if I have tried treating the pain (No)

Q is for **Quality**:

_____Asked me if pain is sharp, dull, crushing, or achy (The pain is sharp)

R is for **Radiation**:

_____Asked where the pain is located (Under my ribs on the right)
_____Asked me if the pain travels anywhere (Yes, my back hurts too)

S is for **Severity**:

_____Asked me to rate the pain on a scale of 1–10, 10 being the worst (The pain is 7/10)

T is for **Time**:

_____Asked how long I have had the pain (About 3 hours)
_____Asked if I have had the pain before (Yes, one other time, but never this bad)
_____Asked if I am still having the pain (Yes)
_____Asked if the pain is constant of intermittent (Constant)

VINDICATE

Vascular:

_____Asked if I vomited blood (No)

Infectious:

_____Asked if I have had a fever or chills (No)
_____Asked if I have had diarrhea (No)
_____Asked about recent travel (No)

Neoplastic: Not applicable

Degenerative: Not applicable

Immunologic: Not applicable

Congenital: Not applicable

(**A**dded) Toxin/poison/drugs:

_____Asked if I use alcohol (I have 2 drinks per day)

Trauma:

_____Asked about an injury to the abdomen (No)

CASE 20 (continued)

Electrolytes/metabolic:

_____Asked about diet (I eat mostly fast food)

Other history:

Past medical history, family history, social history, medication, and allergies: Noncontributory

Review of systems: No headache, chest pain, shortness of breath, diarrhea, or constipation.

Physical Exam Checklist:

_____Washed hands before the exam
_____Asked to untie gown

Head and neck: Not applicable

Chest: Not applicable

Abdomen:

_____Observed abdomen for distention (No distention)
_____Palpated lightly and deeply in all quadrants (Right upper quadrant pain with deep palpation, normal sized liver and spleen, no masses)
_____Asked me to take a deep breath while palpating right upper quadrant (Pain is elicited)
_____Percussed abdomen in all quadrants (Resonant throughout)
_____Listened to abdomen in all quadrants (Active bowel sounds)

Pelvis: Not applicable

Extremities: Not applicable

Skin:

_____Observed skin over abdomen (No lesions)

Nerves: Not applicable

Psychiatric: Not applicable

You should have gotten at least 18 of the 25 possible checkmarks.

CASE 20 (continued)

YOUR NOTE

Differential Diagnosis (list up to 5 in order of likelihood)

1.

2.

3.

4.

5.

History (including positives and negatives from history of present illness, past medical history, family history, social history, and review of systems)

_____

_____

_____

_____

_____

_____

Physical Exam (consisting of positives and negatives relevant to the chief complaint)

_____

_____

_____

_____

_____

_____

Diagnostic Workup (up to 5 items necessary for further diagnosis)

1.

2.

3.

4.

5.

(see p. 140 for sample note)

Sample Notes

CASE 1 (p. 39)

Differential Diagnosis (list up to 5 in order of likelihood)

1. *Tuberculosis*

2. *Pneumonia*

3. *Bronchiectasis*

4. *Lung cancer*

5. *COPD*

History (including positives and negatives from history of present illness, past medical history, family history, social history, and review of systems)

Mr. Davis is a 47-year-old male presenting with a cough that started 1 month ago. The cough is productive of blood-tinged sputum, and worse with physical activity. It has not improved with cold medicine. He is not short of breath, but the cough keeps him up at night. He works in a homeless shelter where he is exposed to tuberculosis. His last PPD was 1 year ago, and it was negative. He does not smoke. He reports having fevers, chills, night sweats, and a 10-pound weight loss. He denies a headache, sore throat, chest pain, shortness of breath, nausea, vomiting, diarrhea, constipation, malaise or lethargy. His past medical history, family history, and social history are noncontributory. He takes no medications and has no allergies.

Physical Exam (consisting of positives and negatives relevant to the chief complaint)

Thin male with a cough. No respiratory distress. Temperature is 100.1°F. All other vitals are normal. No enlarged cervical/supraclavicular lymph nodes. Chest expands symmetrically without dullness to percussion. Lungs clear to auscultation. Heart with regular rate and rhythm. No digital clubbing. Skin is without lesions.

Diagnostic Workup (up to 5 items necessary for further diagnosis)

1. *Chest x-ray*

2. *PPD*

3. *Sputum for Gram stain, acid fast stain, and culture*

4. *HIV test*

5.

CASE 2 (p. 43)

Differential Diagnosis (list up to 5 in order of likelihood)

1. *Viral gastroenteritis*

2. *Bacterial gastroenteritis*

3. *Parasitic gastroenteritis*

4. *Irritable bowel syndrome*

5. *Dietary irritant*

History (including positives and negatives from history of present illness, past medical history, family history, social history, and review of systems)

Ms. Smith is a 27-year-old female presenting with diarrhea and abdominal cramping that started 3 days ago. The diarrhea occurs about 8 times per day, is watery, worse with meals, and minimally responsive to Loperamide. Stool is not bloody, black, or foul smelling. She works in a daycare with numerous sick contacts. She reports having low-grade fevers and a 7-pound weight loss. She denies previous thyroid disease, recent antibiotic use, lactose or gluten sensitivity, or unusual dietary habits. She is not sexually active and denies laxative use. She reports associated nausea and fatigue, but no headache, sore throat, chest pain, shortness of breath, or vomiting. Her past medical history and family history are noncontributory. She has no allergies.

Physical Exam (consisting of positives and negatives relevant to the chief complaint)

Ill-appearing female with no acute distress. Temperature is 100.0°F. All other vital signs are normal. Thyroid is without nodules or enlargement. Abdomen is slightly distended and diffusely tender to deep palpation. No abdominal masses are present. Bowel sounds are hyperactive. Skin is without lesions.

Diagnostic Workup (up to 5 items necessary for further diagnosis)

1. *Rectal exam*

2. *Basic chemistry*

3. *Fecal leukocytes*

4. *Stool culture*

5. *Stool ova and parasite examination*

CASE 3 (p. 47)

Differential Diagnosis (list up to 5 in order of likelihood)

1. *Acute appendicitis*
2. *Ovarian cyst*
3. *Ovarian torsion*
4. *Kidney stones*
5. *Pelvic inflammatory disease*

History (including positives and negatives from history of present illness, past medical history, family history, social history, and review of systems)

Ms. Anderson is a 26-year-old female presenting with sharp, right-sided abdominal pain that started 10 hours ago. The pain is 7/10 in severity. It was originally diffuse and became localized to the lower right side. The pain is made worse with movement. Her last bowel movement was 2 days ago and regular. She has nausea, vomited once, and has no appetite. Her last menstrual period was 2 weeks ago and regular. She is not sexually active and has had no prior surgeries or sexually transmitted diseases. She denies headaches, diarrhea, constipation, dysuria, hematuria, urinary pain/frequency, vaginal discharge, fatigue, and weight loss. Past medical history and family history are noncontributory. She takes no medication and has no allergies.

Physical Exam (consisting of positives and negatives relevant to the chief complaint)

Healthy appearing female with severe right-sided abdominal pain. Temperature is 99.9°F. All other vital signs are normal. Abdomen is slightly distended. Abdominal pain with light palpation, rebound tenderness, and significant muscular resistance to the exam. No abdominal masses are present. Liver and spleen are not enlarged. Hypoactive bowel sounds. Negative psoas sign, positive obturator sign. Skin is without lesions or scars.

Diagnostic Workup (up to 5 items necessary for further diagnosis)

1. *Rectal exam*
2. *Pelvic exam*
3. *Urinalysis*
4. *Complete blood count*
5. *Abdominal/pelvic ultrasound*

CASE 4 (p. 51)

Differential Diagnosis (list up to 5 in order of likelihood)

1. *Myocardial infarction*

2. *Angina*

3. *Aortic dissection*

4. *Pulmonary embolism*

5. *Myocarditis/pericarditis*

History (including positives and negatives from history of present illness, past medical history, family history, social history, and review of systems)

Mr. Clark is a 64-year-old male presenting urgently with crushing, substernal chest pain that radiates to the jaw. The pain is 7/10 in severity. The pain began 4 hours ago while he was mowing the lawn. The pain is made worse with physical activity. He has had pain like this before that was relieved with rest. Rest and aspirin have not helped his current pain. The pain is not related to meals, and he is not short of breath at rest. He has no history of high cholesterol or diabetes. He has a history of hypertension and smoking and a family history of heart disease. He takes no medications and has no allergies. He is nauseated and diaphoretic, but denies fever, chills, weight loss, headache, fainting, lightheadedness, vomiting, diarrhea, constipation, malaise, or fatigue.

Physical Exam (consisting of positives and negatives relevant to the chief complaint)

Diaphoretic, moderately overweight male in obvious discomfort. Blood pressure 150/92, pulse 88. All other vitals signs are normal. Audible carotid bruits bilaterally. Heart is enlarged with a regular rate and rhythm. Chest is symmetric. Lungs are resonant and clear to auscultation. Skin is without lesions or scars.

Diagnostic Workup (up to 5 items necessary for further diagnosis)

1. *ECG*

2. *Chest x-ray*

3. *Cardiac enzymes*

4. *Arterial blood gas*

5. *D-dimer*

CASE 5 (p. 55)

Differential Diagnosis (list up to 5 in order of likelihood)

1. Osteoarthritis
2. Bursitis/tendonitis
3. Rheumatoid arthritis
4. Lyme disease
5. Gout

History (including positives and negatives from history of present illness, past medical history, family history, social history, and review of systems)

Mr. Fisher is a 57-year-old male presenting with knee and hip pain. The pain is dull, worse on the right side, and 5/10 in severity. The pain is worse with physical activity and relived somewhat with ibuprofen. He has morning joint stiffness. He is a retired construction worker and reports frequent minor joint trauma on the job. The pain has worsened over the last few months and now limits his mobility. The patient denies fever or chills, rash, other joint pain, trauma, headaches, chest pain, shortness of breath, nausea, vomiting, diarrhea, constipation, weight loss, malaise, or lethargy. No history of gout or Lyme disease. Family history and social history are noncontributory. He takes no medications and has no allergies.

Physical Exam (consisting of positives and negatives relevant to the chief complaint)

Overweight male in no acute distress. Vital signs are normal. Mild bilateral knee tenderness with firm palpation. Crepitus in knees and hips bilaterally. Limited adduction, abduction, extension, flexion, internal rotation, and external rotation of hips. Limited flexion and extension of knees. Antalgic gait favoring left leg. Bilateral quadriceps and gluteal atrophy. No joint redness, swelling, or warmth.

Diagnostic Workup (up to 5 items necessary for further diagnosis)

1. Erythrocyte sedimentation rate
2. Rheumatoid factor
3. Complete blood count
4. Serum uric acid
5. Lyme titer

CASE 6 (p. 59)

Differential Diagnosis (list up to 5 in order of likelihood)

1. *Bacterial pneumonia*

2. *Atypical pneumonia*

3. *Tuberculosis*

4. *Pulmonary embolism*

5. *COPD*

History (including positives and negatives from history of present illness, past medical history, family history, social history, and review of systems)

Mr. Miller is a 60-year-old male presenting with a cough, fever, and chills that began 3 days ago. He is not short of breath. The cough is constant and productive of yellow sputum. Sputum is never bloody. The cough is not associated with meals or lying down. His symptoms have not improved with cold medicine. He has missed 3 days of work due to his symptoms. He does not smoke. He reports feeling tired and ill lately, but denies chest pain, shortness of breath, nausea, vomiting, diarrhea, constipation, or headache. His past medical history, family history, and social history are noncontributory. He takes no medications and has no allergies.

Physical Exam (consisting of positives and negatives relevant to the chief complaint)

Ill-appearing male with fever and cough without respiratory distress. Temperature is 102.0°F. All other vitals are normal. No enlarged cervical/supraclavicular lymph nodes. Chest is symmetric. Dullness to percussion over left lower lobe. Crackles present diffusely and decreased breath sounds in left lower lobe. Heart with regular rate and rhythm. Skin is without lesions or scars.

Diagnostic Workup (up to 5 items necessary for further diagnosis)

1. *Compete blood count*

2. *Chest x-ray*

3. *Sputum for Gram stain, acid fast stain, and culture*

4. *Arterial blood gases*

5.

CASE 7 (p. 63)

Differential Diagnosis (list up to 5 in order of likelihood)

1. *Stroke*
2. *Transient ischemic attack*
3. *Neoplasm*
4. *Intracranial hemorrhage*
5. *Toxic exposure*

History (including positives and negatives from history of present illness, past medical history, family history, social history, and review of systems)

Mrs. Jacobson is a 76-year-old female brought in urgently by her husband for confusion and inability to move her left arm and leg. She seems unaware of the problem and her husband helped with the history. The symptoms came on gradually about 3 hours ago. She started out confused and then began to lose strength in her leg. Her symptoms appear to be progressing. Past medical history is significant for smoking, hypertension, atherosclerosis, hyperlipidemia, and one myocardial infarct that occurred years ago. She denies headaches, stiff neck, fever, chills, weight loss, seizures, loss of consciousness, chest pain, shortness of breath, nausea, vomiting, diarrhea, or constipation. No history of head trauma or toxic exposures. No family history of Alzheimer's disease. She takes a "cholesterol medication" and has no allergies.

Physical Exam (consisting of positives and negatives relevant to the chief complaint)

Alert female with no acute distress. Blood pressure 156/98. All other vitals are normal. No evidence of head trauma. Lungs clear to auscultation. Heart with regular rate and rhythm. Homonymous hemianopia. No right visual gaze. Pupils equally round and reactive to light. Symmetric facial sensation and muscle strength. Symmetric trapezius and sternocleidomastoid muscle strength. Adequate uvula and tongue movement. Flaccid paralysis of right arm and leg. Reduced light touch sensation in the right hand and foot. Adequate alternating finger to nose test. Brisk right-sided deep tendon reflexes. Positive Babinski sign. Strength, reflexes, and sensation intact on left side. Alert and oriented to place only. Patient unable to perform mental status exam.

Diagnostic Workup (up to 5 items necessary for further diagnosis)

1. *Head CT scan*
2. *Basic chemistry*
3. *Compete blood count*
4. *Prothrombin time (PT)/Partial thromboplastin time (PTT)*
5. *ECG*

CASE 8 (p. 67)

Differential Diagnosis (list up to 5 in order of likelihood)

1. *Lower urinary tract infection*

2. *Vaginitis*

3. *Urethritis*

4. *External irritant (tampon, contraceptive)*

5. *Nephrolithiasis*

History (including positives and negatives from history of present illness, past medical history, family history, social history, and review of systems)

Ms. Nelson is a 22-year-old female presenting with suprapubic pain and burning with urination. She reports having prior urinary tract infections. The pain came on gradually about 3 days ago. The pain is 5/10 in severity. She is sexually active with one partner and uses an oral contraceptive. Her last menstrual period was 2 weeks ago and regular. She denies fevers or chills, headaches, chest pain, shortness of breath, hematuria, vaginal discharge, itching, odor, blistering, diarrhea, constipation, recent trauma, or kidney stones. Past medical history and family history are noncontributory. She has no allergies.

Physical Exam (consisting of positives and negatives relevant to the chief complaint)

Healthy appearing female in no acute distress. Temperature 100°F. All other vital signs are normal. Mild suprapubic tenderness with deep palpation. Normal sized liver and spleen. No palpable abdominal masses. Active bowel sounds. Skin is without lesions or scars.

Diagnostic Workup (up to 5 items necessary for further diagnosis)

1. *Pelvic exam*

2. *Urinalysis*

3. *Urine Gram stain and culture*

4. *KOH preparation*

5. *DNA probe for gonorrhea and chlamydia*

CASE 9 (p. 71)

Differential Diagnosis (list up to 5 in order of likelihood)

1. *Asthma*

2. *Bronchiolitis*

3. *Atypical pneumonia*

4. *Pneumothorax*

5. *Tumor*

History (including positives and negatives from history of present illness, past medical history, family history, social history, and review of systems)

Mr. Daniels is a 21-year-old male presenting with a cough, shortness of breath, and chest tightness that occur intermittently. He is currently short of breath. The symptoms are made worse with exercise, and he is asymptomatic between bouts. He has had similar but less severe symptoms since childhood. He does not smoke. He has seasonal allergies. He denies prior blood clots, prolonged immobility, fever or chills, weight loss or fatigue, toxic exposure including carbon monoxide, aspiration, or trauma to the chest wall. He takes no medications. He denies headaches, sore throat, chest pain, nausea, vomiting, diarrhea, constipation, malaise, or lethargy. His past medical history, family history, and social history are noncontributory.

Physical Exam (consisting of positives and negatives relevant to the chief complaint)

Young adult male with labored breathing. Respiratory rate 24. All other vital signs are normal. No enlarged cervical/supraclavicular lymph nodes. Posterior pharynx is without erythema or lesions. Chest expands symmetrically without dullness to percussion. Tachypnea with diffuse expiratory wheezes. Heart with regular rate and rhythm. Skin is without lesions or scars.

Diagnostic Workup (up to 5 items necessary for further diagnosis)

1. *Arterial blood gas*

2. *Complete blood count*

3. *Pulmonary function tests*

4. *Chest x-ray*

5. *Sputum for Gram stain and culture*

CASE 10 (p. 75)

Differential Diagnosis (list up to 5 in order of likelihood)

1. *Viral hepatitis*
2. *Infectious mononucleosis*
3. *Cholecystitis*
4. *Toxic exposure*
5. *Hemolytic anemia*

History (including positives and negatives from history of present illness, past medical history, family history, social history, and review of systems)

Ms. Becker is a 21-year-old college student presenting with loss of appetite, weakness, jaundice, and pruritis about 3 weeks after travelling in Mexico. The symptoms came on gradually about 1 week ago. She also reports having a fever and chills, diarrhea, crampy abdominal pain, nausea, and an 8-pound weight loss. She is not light-headed or fatigued. She denies dark colored urine or recent blood transfusions. She denies known toxic exposures. She drinks 2 alcoholic drinks per day. She has not received hepatitis vaccinations. She is sexually active with one partner and uses an oral contraceptive for birth control. She denies headaches, chest pain, or shortness of breath. Past medical history and family history are noncontributory. She has no allergies.

Physical Exam (consisting of positives and negatives relevant to the chief complaint)

Ill-appearing female with jaundice. Temperature is 100.2°F. All other vital signs are normal. No enlarged cervical/supraclavicular lymph nodes. Lungs clear to auscultation. Heart with regular rate and rhythm. Liver is enlarged and tender. Mild diffuse abdominal pain. No palpable abdominal masses. Hyperactive bowel sounds. No rashes.

Diagnostic Workup (up to 5 items necessary for further diagnosis)

1. *Compete blood count*
2. *Liver function tests including bilirubin*
3. *Hepatitis serology*
4. *Monospot test for Epstein Barr virus*
5. *Urinalysis*

CASE 11 (p. 79)

Differential Diagnosis (list up to 5 in order of likelihood)

1. *Classic migraine headache*
2. *Tension headache*
3. *Cluster headache*
4. *Sinusitis*
5. *Depression*

History (including positives and negatives from history of present illness, past medical history, family history, social history, and review of systems)

Mr. Andrews is a 31-year-old male complaining of headaches. He does not have a headache now, but his last one was 2 days ago. The headaches begin as a dull throbbing behind the eyes and progress to a sharp pain rated at 9/10 in severity. The patient describes a visual aura. Stress makes them come on, and bright lights, rapid head movements, and coughing make them worse. NSAIDs, sleep, and darkness alleviate the symptoms. The patient had his first headache about 6 months ago and they occur about once every month. The headaches last from a few hours to a day at a time. The patient denies any other neurological symptoms, fever or chills, seizures, trauma, or toxic exposures including drugs, alcohol, and carbon monoxide. He has no sore throat, fever, chills, chest pain, shortness of breath, nausea, vomiting, diarrhea, or constipation. His past medical history and social history are noncontributory. There is a family history of headaches. He takes no medications and has no allergies.

Physical Exam (consisting of positives and negatives relevant to the chief complaint)

Healthy appearing male in no acute distress. All vital signs are normal. No evidence of head trauma. Neck supple. Lungs clear to auscultation. Heart with regular rate and rhythm. Vision adequate, pupils equally round and reactive to light, extraocular muscles intact, symmetric facial sensation and muscle strength, symmetric trapezius and sternocleidomastoid muscle strength, adequate uvula and tongue movement. Adequate and symmetric strength in all extremities. No gait abnormalities, adequate alternating finger to nose test. Reflexes adequate and symmetric. No deficiencies in attention, orientation, memory, abstract thinking, following commands, language usage, or problem solving. No depression.

Diagnostic Workup (up to 5 items necessary for further diagnosis)

1. *Funduscopic exam*
2. *Complete blood count*
3. *Basic chemistry*
4.
5.

CASE 12 (p. 83)

Differential Diagnosis (list up to 5 in order of likelihood)

1. *Cervical neoplasm*
2. *Uterine neoplasm*
3. *Cervical polyps*
4. *Atrophic vaginitis*
5. *Trauma*

History (including positives and negatives from history of present illness, past medical history, family history, social history, and review of systems)

Mrs. Jackson is a 54-year-old G4 P4 female without regular medical care presenting for painless postcoital spotting that began 5 months ago. She reports mild bleeding that occurs only after sex and an occasional yellow, foul smelling vaginal discharge. Menopause was 4 years ago at age 50. She has not had a Pap smear for years, and reports having prior abnormal Pap smears. She is sexually active only with her husband of 30 years. She reports no unusual sexual practices or prior sexually transmitted diseases. She denies headache, chest pain, shortness of breath, nausea, vomiting, diarrhea, constipation, vaginal itching, fatigue, or weight loss. Past medical history and family history are noncontributory. She takes no medications and has no allergies.

Physical Exam (consisting of positives and negatives relevant to the chief complaint)

Moderately overweight female in no acute distress. Vital signs are normal. Lungs are clear to auscultation. Heart with regular rate and rhythm. Liver and spleen are not enlarged. Abdomen is nontender and no masses are present. Active bowel sounds. Multiple matted immobile inguinal lymph nodes are palpable. Skin is without bruises or other lesions.

Diagnostic Workup (up to 5 items necessary for further diagnosis)

1. *Pelvic exam*
2. *Rectal exam*
3. *Pap smear*
4. *Colposcopy and endocervical curettage*
5. *Pelvic ultrasound*

CASE 13 (p. 87)

Differential Diagnosis (list up to 5 in order of likelihood)

1. *Placenta previa*

2. *Placental abruption*

3. *Preterm labor*

4. *Trauma*

5. *Coagulation disorder*

History (including positives and negatives from history of present illness, past medical history, family history, social history, and review of systems)

Mrs. Evans is a 24-year-old G2 P1 female at 31 weeks gestation presenting with painless vaginal bleeding that began about 2 weeks ago after sexual intercourse. The blood is bight red with some clots. The bleeding was light at first, but has increased and now occurs almost daily. She is not lightheaded or more fatigued than usual for her pregnancy. She denies prior sexually transmitted diseases, bleeding problems, vaginal discharge, fever or chills, trauma, pain with urination, alcohol or drug use, headaches, chest pain, shortness of breath, nausea, vomiting, diarrhea, or constipation. Past medical history and family history are noncontributory. She takes prenatal vitamins and has no allergies.

Physical Exam (consisting of positives and negatives relevant to the chief complaint)

Healthy appearing pregnant female in no acute distress. Vital signs are normal. Fetal heart rate is 140. Lungs are clear to auscultation. Heart with regular rate and rhythm. Gravid uterus with size consistent with gestational age. Fetus is longitudinal and cephalic. Liver and spleen are not enlarged. No abdominal tenderness or masses. Bowel sounds are active. Skin is without lesions.

Diagnostic Workup (up to 5 items necessary for further diagnosis)

1. *Pelvic ultrasound*

2. *Pelvic exam*

3. *Complete blood count*

4. *Protime (PT)*

5. *Partial thromboplastin time (PTT)*

CASE 14 (p. 91)

Differential Diagnosis (list up to 5 in order of likelihood)

1. Gout

2. Pseudogout

3. Septic arthritis

4. Osteomyelitis

5. Lyme disease

History (including positives and negatives from history of present illness, past medical history, family history, social history, and review of systems)

Mr. Jensen is a 60-year-old male presenting with severe left toe and foot pain. The pain is crushing, constant, and 10/10 in severity. It began in his big toe and now involves the whole foot. He has had the pain for about 1 day. He gets no relief from NSAIDs. The patient denies prior blood clots, vascular disease, rash, other joint pain, trauma, headaches, chest pain, shortness of breath, nausea, vomiting, diarrhea, constipation, or weight loss. Past medical history, family history, and social history are noncontributory. He takes no medications and has no allergies.

Physical Exam (consisting of positives and negatives relevant to the chief complaint)

Obese male with severe left toe and foot tenderness. Temperature is 101.0° F. All other vital signs are normal. Lungs are clear to auscultation. Heart with regular rate and rhythm. Left toe and foot are red and swollen with tense, shiny skin. All other joints are nontender with adequate range of motion. Skin is without rashes or other lesions.

Diagnostic Workup (up to 5 items necessary for further diagnosis)

1. Serum uric acid

2. Joint aspiration

3. Crystal analysis, culture, and gram stain of synovial fluid

4. Complete blood count

5. Basic chemistry

CASE 15 (p. 95)

Differential Diagnosis (list up to 5 in order of likelihood)

1. *Prostatic hypertrophy*
2. *Prostate cancer*
3. *Prostatitis*
4. *Urinary tract infection*
5. *Nephrolithiasis*

History (including positives and negatives from history of present illness, past medical history, family history, social history, and review of systems)

Mr. Watson is a 72-year-old male presenting with nocturia and urinary urgency, frequency, and hesitancy that began 6 weeks ago. His symptoms are worse with increased fluid intake. He is able to empty his bladder with straining. His last prostate exam was years ago and the results are unknown. He drinks 1 cup of coffee per day and takes no alcohol, diuretics, or herbal supplements. He is not sexually active now and has no history of sexually transmitted diseases. He denies hematuria, dysuria, and bladder or bowel incontinence. Review of systems negative for fever, chills, headache, chest pain, shortness of breath, nausea, vomiting, diarrhea, constipation, fatigue, or weight loss. Past medical history and family history are noncontributory. He takes no medications and has no allergies.

Physical Exam (consisting of positives and negatives relevant to the chief complaint)

Moderately overweight male in no acute distress. Vital signs are normal. Abdomen is nontender. Bladder dome is palpable. Liver and spleen are not enlarged. No abdominal masses are present. Bowel sounds are active. Strength and sensation are adequate and symmetric in both legs. Skin is without lesions.

Diagnostic Workup (up to 5 items necessary for further diagnosis)

1. *Rectal exam*
2. *Urinalysis*
3. *Basic chemistry*
4. *Complete blood count*
5. *Prostate specific antigen (PSA)*

CASE 16 (p. 99)

Differential Diagnosis (list up to 5 in order of likelihood)

1. *Venous thrombosis*

2. *Cellulitis*

3. *Hematoma*

4. *Compartment syndrome*

5. *Ruptured popliteal (Baker's) cyst*

History (including positives and negatives from history of present illness, past medical history, family history, social history, and review of systems)

Mr. Huggins is a 36-year-old male complaining of pain and swelling in his left lower leg. He is a long-distance truck driver who first noticed the pain 1 day ago after driving for about 5 hours straight. He describes the pain as a tight, pressure sensation that is 4/10 in severity and made worse by walking. The symptoms are constant and seem to be getting worse. He smokes 1 pack per day and often sits for long periods of time. He denies leg trauma, chest pain, shortness of breath, a cancer history, and a personal or family history of blood clots. He has no headache, fever, chills, nausea, vomiting, diarrhea, or constipation. Past medical history and social history are noncontributory. He takes no medications and has no allergies.

Physical Exam (consisting of positives and negatives relevant to the chief complaint)

Healthy appearing male with no acute distress. Vital signs are normal. Lungs are clear to auscultation bilaterally. Heart with regular rate and rhythm. Left leg is warm, tender, erythematous, and swollen from toe to knee. There is moderate pitting edema. Pain with dorsiflexion of the left calf. Strong palpable dorsalis pedis pulses bilaterally. Right leg is not swollen, tender, or erythematous.

Diagnostic Workup (up to 5 items necessary for further diagnosis)

1. *Lower leg Doppler ultrasound*

2. *Compete blood count*

3. *Prothrombin time (PT) and Partial thromboplastin time (PTT)*

4.

5.

CASE 17 (p. 103)

Differential Diagnosis (list up to 5 in order of likelihood)

1. *Peptic ulcer disease*
2. *Gastritis*
3. *Gastroesophageal reflux*
4. *Pancreatitis*
5. *Neoplasm*

History (including positives and negatives from history of present illness, past medical history, family history, social history, and review of systems)

Mr. Thomas is a 52-year-old male complaining of burning chest pain over the last month. The pain is in his lower chest/midepigastic region, intermittent, and 6/10 in severity. It is made worse by alcohol, coffee, and lying down at night. It is somewhat improved by antacids and light bland meals. He has had occasional dark stools. No hematemesis, light-headedness, or fatigue. He smokes a half pack per day and drinks about 3 alcoholic drinks per night. He takes NSAIDs frequently for arthritis. He denies headaches, shortness of breath, fever or chills, nausea, vomiting, diarrhea, or constipation. Past medical history, family history, and social history are noncontributory. He takes no medications (except NSAIDs) and has no allergies.

Physical Exam (consisting of positives and negatives relevant to the chief complaint)

Healthy appearing male in no acute distress. All vital signs are normal. Lungs are clear to auscultation. Heart with regular rate and rhythm. Mild midepigastric tenderness with deep palpation. Liver and spleen are not enlarged. No palpable masses. Active bowel sounds. Skin is without lesions.

Diagnostic Workup (up to 5 items necessary for further diagnosis)

1. *Complete blood count*
2. *Basic chemistry*
3. *Amylase/lipase*
4. *Upper endoscopy*
5. *Helicobacter pylori serology*

CASE 18 (p. 107)

Differential Diagnosis (list up to 5 in order of likelihood)

1. Sprain

2. Herniated disc

3. Osteoarthritis

4. Lumbar spinal stenosis

5. Tumor

History (including positives and negatives from history of present illness, past medical history, family history, social history, and review of systems)

Mr. Thompson is a 45-year-old male complaining of dull, achy low back pain that is sometimes associated with left lower leg weakness and numbness. The pain is constant and located centrally in his lower lumbar area. It became acutely worse yesterday after some heavy lifting. The pain is made worse with lifting, sudden movements, and prolonged sitting. Aspirin gives some relief. He denies loss of bowel or bladder function, fever or chills, arthritis, other joint pain, trauma, or previous tumors. He denies headaches, chest pain, shortness of breath, nausea, vomiting, diarrhea, or constipation. Past medical history, family history, and social history are noncontributory. He takes no medications and has no allergies.

Physical Exam (consisting of positives and negatives relevant to the chief complaint)

Healthy appearing male in no acute distress. Vital signs are normal. Lungs are clear to auscultation bilaterally. Heart with regular rate and rhythm. Legs are symmetric without muscle atrophy. Low back pain with bending backward. Lumbar range of motion otherwise adequate. Light touch sensation and plantar flexion strength is diminished in the left foot. No gait abnormalities. Reflexes are adequate and symmetric.

Diagnostic Workup (up to 5 items necessary for further diagnosis)

1. No further testing is necessary

2.

3.

4.

5.

CASE 19 (p. 111)

Differential Diagnosis (list up to 5 in order of likelihood)

1. *Ectopic pregnancy*
2. *Threatened abortion*
3. *Pelvic inflammatory disease*
4. *Endometriosis*
5. *Ovarian cyst*

History (including positives and negatives from history of present illness, past medical history, family history, social history, and review of systems)

Ms. Baker is a 20-year-old G2 Ab1 female at 8 weeks gestation by last menstrual period complaining of abdominal pain and vaginal bleeding. The pain and bleeding began suddenly about 2 hours ago. The pain is constant, sharp, 6/10 in severity, located in the left pelvis. It radiates to her upper back and shoulders. The blood is bright red and scant. She denies prior bleeding problems, lightheadedness, or fatigue. No fever, chills, vaginal discharge, unusual odor, or urinary symptoms. She last had intercourse 1 week ago, and denies dyspareunia. Has had one sexual partner and engages only in penile-vaginal sex. She had a gonorrhea infection several years ago. Her last menstrual period was 8 weeks ago and regular. She denies headache, fatigue, chest pain, shortness of breath, nausea, vomiting, diarrhea, or constipation.

Physical Exam (consisting of positives and negatives relevant to the chief complaint)

Healthy appearing female with obvious abdominal discomfort. All vital signs are normal. Lungs are clear to auscultation. Heart with regular rate and rhythm. No abdominal distention. Moderate left lower quadrant tenderness with deep palpation. Liver and spleen not enlarged. No palpable abdominal masses. No flank tenderness. Active bowel sounds. No skin lesions or bruises.

Diagnostic Workup (up to 5 items necessary for further diagnosis)

1. *Pelvic exam*
2. *Quantitative hCG*
3. *Urinalysis*
4. *Complete blood count*
5. *Pelvic ultrasound*

CASE 20 (p. 115)

Differential Diagnosis (list up to 5 in order of likelihood)

1. *Biliary colic*

2. *Cholecystitis*

3. *Cholangitis*

4. *Peptic ulcer disease*

4. *Pancreatitis*

History (including positives and negatives from history of present illness, past medical history, family history, social history, and review of systems)

Mrs. Peterson is a 46-year-old female presenting with 3 hours of nausea, vomiting, and abdominal pain. The pain is constant, sharp, under her ribs on the right, and 7/10 in severity. The pain radiates to her back and is worse with meals. She has had similar pain once before. She denies trauma, hematemesis, fever or chills, diarrhea, or recent travel. She drinks 2 drinks per day and eats mostly fast food. She denies headache, chest pain, shortness of breath, diarrhea, or constipation. Past medical history, family history, and social history are noncontributory. She takes no medication and has no allergies.

Physical Exam (consisting of positives and negatives relevant to the chief complaint)

Diaphoretic, obese female with obvious discomfort. All vital signs are normal. Abdomen is not distended. Right upper quadrant pain with deep palpation, normal sized liver and spleen, no masses. Positive Murphy's sign. Abdomen with resonant percussion. Active bowel sounds. Skin without lesions.

Diagnostic Workup (up to 5 items necessary for further diagnosis)

1. *Abdominal ultrasound*

2. *Serum bilirubin*

3. *Alkaline phosphatase*

4. *Complete blood count*

5. *Amylase/lipase*

References

1. Tombleson P, Fox RA, Dacre JA. Defining the content for the objective structured clinical examination component of the professional and linguistic assessments board examination: development of a blueprint. Med Educ 2000;34:566–572.

2. United States Medical Licensing Examination Website. Available at: http://www.usmle.org. Accessed April 14, 2004.

3. Tamblyn RM, Klass DJ, Schnabl GK, Kopelow ML. The accuracy of standardized patient presentation. Med Educ 1991;25:100–109.

4. Newble, D. Techniques for measuring clinical competence: objective structured clinical examinations. Med Educ 2004;38:199–203.

5. Cusimano, MD. Standard setting in medical education. Acad Med 1996;71 (suppl):S112–120.

6. Kaufman DM, Mann KV, Muijtjens AN, van der Vleuten CP. A comparison of standard-setting procedures for an OSCE in undergraduate medical education. Acad Med 2000;75:267–271.

Index

Index note: page references in **bold** indicate discussion of subject in practice case sample answers.

Abdominal cramping, 43–46, **122**

Abdominal pain, 19, 47–50, 111–114, 115–118, **123, 139, 140**

Abortion, threatened, as differential dx, **139**

Acute appendicitis, as differential dx, **123**

Alcohol abuse, 29

Allergies, as checklist item, 15

Angina, as differential dx, **124**

Angoff scoring method, 35–36

Aortic dissection, as differential dx, **124**

Appetite, loss of, 43–46, **122**

Asthma, as differential dx, **129**

Atrophic vaginitis, as differential dx, **132**

Atypical cases, 27–30

Atypical pneumonia, as differential dx, **126, 129**

Auscultation, 18

Back pain, lower, 107–110, **138**

Bacterial gastroenteritis, as differential dx, **122**

Bacterial pneumonia, as differential dx, **126**

Bad news, communication of, 19, 27–28

Behavior changes, assessment of, 28–29

Biliary colic, as differential dx, **140**

Bleeding, postcoital, 83–86, **132**

Body regions, 11

Borderline scoring method, 35–36

Bronchiectasis, as differential dx, **121**

Bronchiolitis, as differential dx, **129**

Burning chest pain, 103–106, **137**

Cellulitis, as differential dx, **136**

Cervical neoplasm, as differential dx, **132**

Cervical polyps, as differential dx, **132**

Checklists
  changing sequence of, 33
  items on, 14, 15
  PQRST checklist in, 13–14, 24, 25, 28, 37
  in practice cases, 37, 39–121
  in scoring methods, 34–36
  VINDICATE checklist in, 11, 13–14, 24, 25, 28, 37

Chest pain, 19, 51–54, 103–106, **124, 137**

Chest tightness, 71–74, **129**

Cholangitis, as differential dx, **140**

Cholecystitis, as differential dx, **130, 140**

Chronic obstructive pulmonary disease (COPD), as differential dx, **121, 126**

Classic migraine headache, as differential dx, **131**

Clinical Skills Assessment (CSA), xiii

Cluster headache, as differential dx, **131**

Coagulation disorder, as differential dx, **133**

Communication/communication skills
  in atypical cases, 27–30
  of bad news, 19, 27–28

Communication/communication
skills (*continued*)
consideration of patient's emotions in,
21
courtesy and professional manners in,
20–23
during history and physical exams,
19–22
spoken English proficiency in, 9, 22–23,
34
style and grace in awkward situations,
31–33
Compartment syndrome, as differential dx,
136
Confusion in mental status, 63–66, **127**
Consent, obtaining, 28
Cough
with chest tightness, 71–74, **129**
with fever, 59–62, **126**
persistent, 39–42, **121**
with shortness of breath, 71–74, **129**
Cut down, Annoyed by criticism, Guilt
about using, Eye opener in the
morning (CAGE) questions, 29

Depression, as differential dx, **131**
Diagnostic workup, 25
Diarrhea, 43–46, **122**
Dietary irritant, as differential dx, **122**
Differential diagnosis
in medical notes, 13–14, 20, 23–24
in practice cases, 39–140

Ectopic pregnancy, as differential dx,
139
Edema/swelling, of lower leg,
99–102, **136**
Endometriosis, as differential dx, **139**
English proficiency, 9, 22–23, 34
Exam
categories of medical complaints in, 4
forming differential diagnosis for, 13–14,
20, 23–24
history and physical exam checklists for,
10–11, 16, 23–26
note taking and writing, 16, 23–25, 26
preparation and warm-up for, 7–9

scoring methods of, 34–36
specific skill levels tested in, 9, 12,
34–36
spoken English proficiency in, 9, 22–23,
34
standardized patients and simulations in,
2, 5–6, 32
structure and process of, 9, 10–26
style and grace with awkward situations,
31–33
testable clinical situations for, 3–4
writing the medical note for, 16, 23–25,
26
Examination blueprints, 3–4
External irritants, as differential dx,
128

Family counseling, 29
Family history, 14
Fever, 59–62, **126**
Flaccid paralysis, 63–66, **127**
Foot pain, 91–94, **134**

Gastritis, as differential dx, **137**
Gastroesophageal reflux, as differential dx,
137
Genetic diseases, 29
Gout, as differential dx, **134**

Headache, 79–82, **131**
Hematoma, as differential dx, **136**
Hemolytic anemia, as differential dx,
130
Herniated disc, as differential dx, **138**
Hip pain, 55–58, **125**
History
body regions and organ systems in, 10,
11–16
complete or focused, 12–16
family history in, 14
hidden findings in, 30
medical history in, 14
PQRST checklist for, 12–13, 24, 25, 28,
37
social history in, 14–15
VINDICATE checklist for, 11, 13–14,
24, 25, 28, 37

Infectious mononucleosis, as differential dx, **130**

Intracranial hemorrhage, as differential dx, **127**

Irritable bowel syndrome, as differential dx, **122**

Jaundice, 75–78, **130**

Joint pain, lower extremities, 55–58, **125**

Kidney stone, as differential dx, **123**

Knee pain, 55–58, **125**

Laboratory results, interpretation of, 30

Leg, pain and swelling of, 99–102, **136**

Lower back pain, 107–110, **138**

Lower extremities, leg pain and swelling, 99–102, **136**

Lumbar spinal stenosis, as differential dx, **138**

Lung cancer, as differential dx, **121**

Lyme disease, as differential dx, **134**

Medical test results, interpretation of, 30

Medications, patient history of, 15

Mental status changes, 28–29, 63–66, **127**

Myocardial infarction, as differential dx, **124**

Myocarditis, as differential dx, **124**

Nausea and vomiting, 115–118, **140**

Neoplasm, as differential dx, **127, 137**

Nephrolithiasis, as differential dx, **128, 135**

Noncompliance, 28

Note writing, 16, 23–25, 26

Objective Structured Clinical Exam (OSCE), xiii

Observation, 17

Organ systems, 11, 15–16

Osteoarthritis, as differential dx, **138**

Osteomyelitis, as differential dx, **134**

Ovarian cyst, as differential dx, **123, 139**

Ovarian torsion, as differential dx, **123**

Palpation, 17

Pancreatitis, as differential dx, **137, 140**

Paralysis, flaccid, 63–66, **127**

Parasitic gastroenteritis, as differential dx, **122**

Patients

atypical cases of, 27–30

courtesy and meeting of, 11–12

examination stations of, 9, 10–26

noncompliant, 28

obtaining a consent from, 28

physical exams of, 16–19

questions asked by, 19, 21–22

refusing treatment by, 28

secret-keeping by, 27

standardized patients as, 2, 5–6

style and grace in awkward situations with, 31–33

taking a history of, 10–11, 12–16

testable clinical situations of, 3–4

See also Communication/communication skills

Pelvic inflammatory disease, as differential dx, **123, 139**

Peptic ulcer disease, as differential dx, **137, 140**

Percussion, 17–18

Pericarditis, as differential dx, **124**

Physical exams

components of, 17–19

prohibited exams in, 16–17

technique of, 18

Placental abruption, as differential dx, **133**

Placenta previa, as differential dx, **133**

Pneumonia, as differential dx, **121, 126, 129**

Pneumothorax, as differential dx, **129**

Popliteal (Baker's) cyst, ruptured, as differential dx, **136**

Practice cases, 37, 39–140

Pregnancy

as checklist item, 14

with vaginal bleeding, 87–90, 111–114, **133, 139**

Preterm labor, as differential dx, **133**

Prostate cancer, as differential dx, **135**

Prostatic hypertrophy, as differential dx, **135**

Prostatitis, as differential dx, **135**

Provokes, Quality, Radiation, Severity, Time (PQRST) checklist, 13–14, 24, 25, 28, 37

Pruritis, 75–78, **130**

Pseudogout, as differential dx, **134**

Psychiatric assessments, 28–29

Pulmonary embolism, as differential dx, **124, 126**

Refusal of treatment, 28

Ruptured popliteal (Baker's) cyst, as differential dx, **136**

Scoring
 Angoff and borderline methods of, 35–36
 checklist method of, 33
 determining pass and fail with, 35–36
 evaluation criteria and methods of, 34–36

Septic arthritis, as differential dx, **134**

Shortness of breath, 19, 35, 71–74, **129**

Sickle cell anemia, 29

Sinusitis, as differential dx, **131**

Skin complaints, 75–78, **130**

Smoking, 29

Social history, 14–15

Spotting, postcoital, 83–86, **132**

Sprain, as differential dx, **138**

Standardized patients, 2, 5–6, 14

Stroke, as differential dx, **127**

Suicidal patients, 29

Swelling, of lower leg, 99–102, **136**

Tension headache, as differential dx, **131**

Tests, interpretation of, 30

Threatened abortion, as differential dx, **139**

Tobacco addiction, 29

Toxic exposure, as differential dx, **127, 130**

Transient ischemic attack, as differential dx, **127**

Trauma, as differential dx, **132, 133**

Tuberculosis, as differential dx, **121, 126**

Tumor, as differential dx, **129, 138**

United States Medical Licensing Examination (USMLE)
 Step 2 Clinical Skills (USMLE Step 2 CS), xiii, 1–2
 website of, xi

Urethritis, as differential dx, **128**

Urinary tract infection, as differential dx, **128, 135**

Urination
 frequency and pain with, 67–70, **128**
 hesitancy with, 95–98, **135**

Uterine neoplasm, as differential dx, **132**

Vaginal bleeding
 postcoital, 83–86, **132**
 pregnancy with, 87–90, 111–114, **133, 139**

Vaginitis, as differential dx, **128, 132**

Vascular, Infectious, Neoplastic, Degenerative, Immunologic, Congenital, Added, Trauma, Electrolytes/metabolic (VINDICATE) checklist, 11, 13–14, 24, 25, 28, 37

Venous thrombosis, as differential dx, **136**

Viral gastroenteritis, as differential dx, **122**

Viral hepatitis, as differential dx, **130**

Weakness, 75–78, **130**

Weight loss, 43–46, **122**